NATIONAL ACADEMIES

Sciences
Engineering
Medicine

NATIONAL
ACADEMIES
PRESS
Washington, DC

Increasing the Utility of Wastewater-based Disease Surveillance for Public Health Action

A Phase 2 Report

Committee on Community
Wastewater-based Infectious
Disease Surveillance

Water Science and Technology
Board

Division on Earth and Life Studies

Board on Population Health and
Public Health Practice

Health and Medicine Division

Consensus Study Report

NATIONAL ACADEMIES PRESS   500 Fifth Street, NW   Washington, DC 20001

This activity was supported by a contract between the National Academy of Sciences and the Centers for Disease Control and Prevention under Contract No. 75D30121D11240 and 75D30123F00017. Any opinions, findings, conclusions, or recommendations expressed in this publication do not necessarily reflect the views of any organization or agency that provided support for the project.

International Standard Book Number-13: 978-0-309-71620-8
International Standard Book Number-10: 0-309-71620-9
Digital Object Identifier: https://doi.org/10.17226/27516
Library of Congress Control Number: 2024949405

This publication is available from the National Academies Press, 500 Fifth Street, NW, Keck 360, Washington, DC 20001; (800) 624-6242 or (202) 334-3313; http://www.nap.edu.

Suggested citation: National Academies of Sciences, Engineering, and Medicine. 2024. *Increasing the Utility of Wastewater-based Disease Surveillance for Public Health Action: A Phase 2 Report*. Washington, DC: The National Academies Press. https://doi.org/10.17226/27516.

The **National Academy of Sciences** was established in 1863 by an Act of Congress, signed by President Lincoln, as a private, nongovernmental institution to advise the nation on issues related to science and technology. Members are elected by their peers for outstanding contributions to research. Dr. Marcia McNutt is president.

The **National Academy of Engineering** was established in 1964 under the charter of the National Academy of Sciences to bring the practices of engineering to advising the nation. Members are elected by their peers for extraordinary contributions to engineering. Dr. John L. Anderson is president.

The **National Academy of Medicine** (formerly the Institute of Medicine) was established in 1970 under the charter of the National Academy of Sciences to advise the nation on medical and health issues. Members are elected by their peers for distinguished contributions to medicine and health. Dr. Victor J. Dzau is president.

The three Academies work together as the **National Academies of Sciences, Engineering, and Medicine** to provide independent, objective analysis and advice to the nation and conduct other activities to solve complex problems and inform public policy decisions. The National Academies also encourage education and research, recognize outstanding contributions to knowledge, and increase public understanding in matters of science, engineering, and medicine.

Learn more about the National Academies of Sciences, Engineering, and Medicine at **www.nationalacademies.org**.

Consensus Study Reports published by the National Academies of Sciences, Engineering, and Medicine document the evidence-based consensus on the study's statement of task by an authoring committee of experts. Reports typically include findings, conclusions, and recommendations based on information gathered by the committee and the committee's deliberations. Each report has been subjected to a rigorous and independent peer-review process and it represents the position of the National Academies on the statement of task.

Proceedings published by the National Academies of Sciences, Engineering, and Medicine chronicle the presentations and discussions at a workshop, symposium, or other event convened by the National Academies. The statements and opinions contained in proceedings are those of the participants and are not endorsed by other participants, the planning committee, or the National Academies.

Rapid Expert Consultations published by the National Academies of Sciences, Engineering, and Medicine are authored by subject-matter experts on narrowly focused topics that can be supported by a body of evidence. The discussions contained in rapid expert consultations are considered those of the authors and do not contain policy recommendations. Rapid expert consultations are reviewed by the institution before release.

For information about other products and activities of the National Academies, please visit www.nationalacademies.org/about/whatwedo.

v

BOARD ON POPULATION HEALTH AND
PUBLIC HEALTH PRACTICE

Reviewers

This Consensus Study Report was reviewed in draft form by individuals chosen for their diverse perspectives and technical expertise. The purpose of this independent review is to provide candid and critical comments that will assist the National Academies of Sciences, Engineering, and Medicine in making each published report as sound as possible and to ensure that it meets the institutional standards for quality, objectivity, evidence, and responsiveness to the study charge. The review comments and draft manuscript remain confidential to protect the integrity of the deliberative process.

We thank the following individuals for their review of this report:

KYLE BIBBY, University of Notre Dame
ALEXANDRIA BOEHM, Stanford University
SARA CODY, Santa Clara County Public Health
MICHAEL DIAMOND, Washington University in St. Louis
JOHN DRAKE, University of Georgia
DANIEL GERRITY, Southern Nevada Water Authority
MICHAEL LAIRMORE, University of California, Davis
JOSHUA LEVY, Scripps Research Institute
AMY MATHERS, University of Virginia
ANNA MEHROTRA, Water Environment Foundation
MIRIAM NUNO, University of California, Davis
KIRSTEN WEISBECK, Colorado Department of Public Health
    and Environment

Although these reviewers provided many constructive comments and suggestions, they were not asked to endorse the conclusions and recommendations, nor did they see the final draft of the report before its release. The review of this report was overseen by **RHODES TRUSSELL (NAE)**, Trussell Technologies Inc., and **GEORGES C. BENJAMIN (NAM)**, American Public Health Association. Appointed by the National Academies, they were responsible for making certain that an independent examination of this report was carried out in accordance with institutional procedures and that all review comments received full consideration. Responsibility for the final content of this report rests entirely with the authoring committee and the National Academies.

Acronyms

APHL	Association of Public Health Laboratories
BSL	biosafety level
CDC	U.S. Centers for Disease Control and Prevention
DCIPHER	Data Collation and Integration for Public Health Event Response
ddPCR	droplet digital polymerase chain reaction
DNA	deoxyribonucleic acid
dPCR	digital polymerase chain reaction
ED	emergency department
EMMI	Environmental Microbiology Minimum Information
EPA	U.S. Environmental Protection Agency
ESBL	extended spectrum β-lactamase
ESSENCE	Electronic Surveillance System for the Early Notification of Community-Based Epidemics
EVD68	enterovirus D68
EWMA	exponentially weighted moving average
HHS	U.S. Department of Health and Human Services
HMPV	human metapneumovirus
HPIV	human parainfluenza
HUS	hemolytic uremic syndrome

ICU	intensive care unit
IIS	Immunization Information System
LODES	Longitudinal Employer-Household Dynamics Origin-Destination Employment Statistics
LOQ	limit of quantitation
LOWESS	locally weighted scatterplot smoothing
MERS-CoV	Middle East respiratory syndrome coronavirus
MIQE	Minimum Information for Publication of Quantitative Real-Time PCR Experiments
MPN	most probable number
MSA	metropolitan statistical area
NEDSS	National Electronic Disease Surveillance System
NIH	National Institutes of Health
NNDSS	National Notifiable Diseases Surveillance System
NSF	National Science Foundation
NSSIL	National Sewage Surveillance Interagency Leadership
NSSP	National Syndromic Surveillance Program
NWSS	National Wastewater Surveillance System
PCR	polymerase chain reaction
PMMoV	pepper mild mottle virus
QA-QC	quality assurance and quality control
qPCR	quantitative polymerase chain reaction
RNA	ribonucleic acid
rRNA	ribosomal ribonucleic acid
RSV	respiratory syncytial virus
RT-PCR	reverse transcription polymerase chain reaction
RT-qPCR	reverse transcription-quantitative polymerase chain reaction
SEIR	Susceptible–Exposed–Infected–Recovered
SOP	standard operating procedure
STEC	Shiga-toxin-producing E. coli
STI	sexually transmitted infection
SVI	Social Vulnerability Index
TSE	transmissible spongiform encephalopathy
TSS	total suspended solids

USDA	U.S. Department of Agriculture
USGS	U.S. Geological Survey
WastewaterSCAN	Sewer Coronavirus Alert Network
WEF	Water Environment Federation
WHO	World Health Organization
WVAL	wastewater viral activity level
WWTP	wastewater treatment plant

Contents

1

Introduction

Wastewater-based infectious disease surveillance describes the ongoing collection, analysis, and interpretation of and response to data related to the transmission of pathogens in wastewater for public health purposes. In wastewater surveillance systems, untreated municipal wastewater is sampled and analyzed for the presence of biomarkers of infection, most commonly pathogen deoxyribonucleic acid (DNA) or ribonucleic acid (RNA) that are shed by infected persons (see Figure 1-1). The measurement is inherently an indicator of the magnitude of the agent's loading to wastewater, which can be interpreted to understand the presence and increases or decreases in prevalence of infection in a community. Wastewater surveillance can capture pre-symptomatic and asymptomatic cases as well as infections across the spectrum of disease severity, regardless of people's care-seeking behavior. During the COVID-19 pandemic, wastewater surveillance gained traction and was implemented rapidly as an additional epidemiological tool to monitor trends and anticipate disease incidence in communities.

Whereas clinical laboratory testing and health services track individual cases of infection, testing for a pathogen at a wastewater treatment plant (also known as community-level wastewater surveillance) provides aggregate data from an entire community sewershed (i.e., the community population consisting of homes, businesses, and other institutions that share a common sewer system or drainage area). It does not track or identify infectious disease for an individual person or household; rather, it detects the presence and changing quantities of a pathogen within the larger community. More focused sampling can take place within the sewershed at manholes or pump stations to capture information about disease in subsets of the population (termed sub-sewershed sampling) or at facilities, such as hospitals or long-term care facilities.

In the United States, 84 percent of households are connected to a wastewater treatment plant (U.S. Census, 2022). The remaining unsewered population is not directly addressed by this epidemiological approach, although some members of this population regularly commute to sewered areas for work, school, or other activities.

WASTEWATER SURVEILLANCE IN THE UNITED STATES

Wastewater surveillance was implemented quickly across the country under emergency conditions during the COVID-19 pandemic, with independent development of many local and hyperlocal (e.g., building- or institution-based) initiatives. As proof-of-concept was established for the feasibility and potential public health value of SARS-CoV-2 RNA detection, the implementation of these systems expanded. Recognizing the need for centralization and coordination of these efforts, the U.S. Centers for Disease Control and Prevention (CDC) launched the National Wastewater Surveillance System (NWSS) in partnership with the U.S. Department of Health and Human Services (HHS) in September 2020. Through the NWSS, CDC coordinates with state-, tribal-, local-, and territorial-level health departments to design and integrate wastewater surveillance data to inform public health decisions.

The NWSS was the first national-level wastewater disease surveillance system in the United States and has been supported by $500 million in pandemic response funding over 4 years. As of April 2024, the NWSS was receiving data from more than 1,300 active sampling sites, covering a population of 130 million individuals (Figure 1-2).[1] This includes data collected through WastewaterSCAN, a privately funded wastewater surveillance initiative with over 180 sites across the nation in 2024.[2] The participation of most other sites is supported by CDC Epidemiology and Laboratory Capacity for Prevention and Control of Emerging Infectious Diseases (ELC) Cooperative Agreement grants provided to eligible health departments (i.e., state health departments, territories, and some large cities and counties). This cooperative agreement extends through fiscal year (FY) 2027.

Wastewater surveillance sampling sites are based in participating municipal wastewater systems; communities and populations that are unsewered are only captured in a wastewater surveillance system to the extent that individuals commute to a monitored sewershed for work, school, or other activities. The sizes of communities in the NWSS served by an individual

---

[1] See https://www.cdc.gov/nwss/about.html.
[2] See https://data.wastewaterscan.org/publications/.

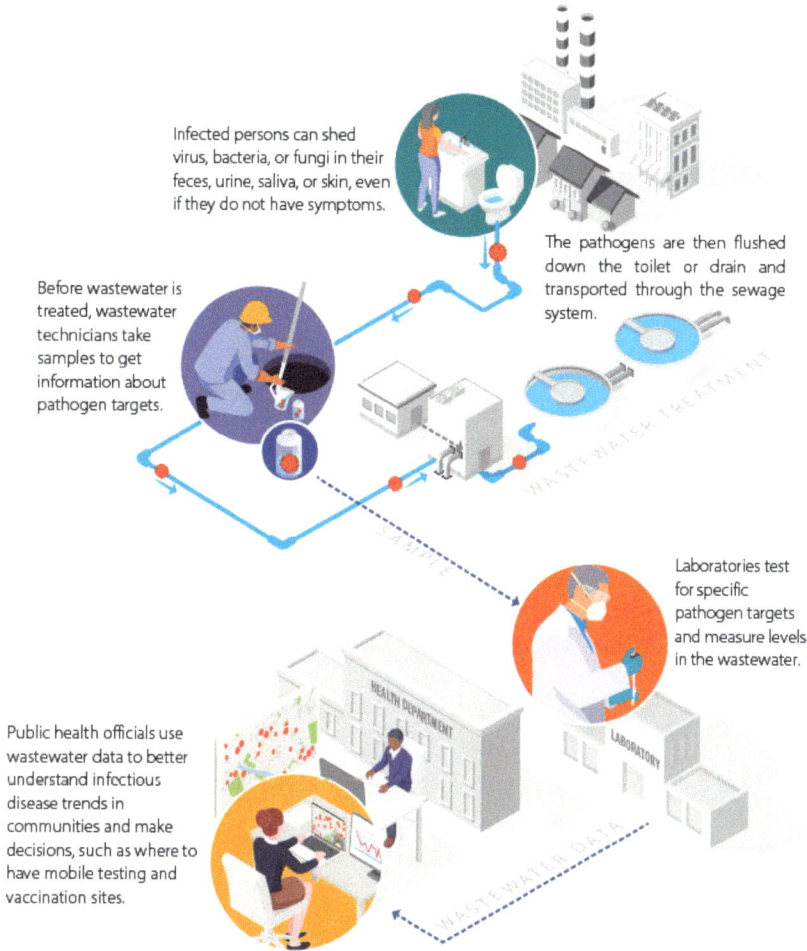

Infected persons can shed virus, bacteria, or fungi in their feces, urine, saliva, or skin, even if they do not have symptoms.

The pathogens are then flushed down the toilet or drain and transported through the sewage system.

Before wastewater is treated, wastewater technicians take samples to get information about pathogen targets.

Laboratories test for specific pathogen targets and measure levels in the wastewater.

Public health officials use wastewater data to better understand infectious disease trends in communities and make decisions, such as where to have mobile testing and vaccination sites.

FIGURE 1-1 Components of a community-level wastewater surveillance system. Infected persons can shed biomarkers of infection (see Box 1-1) into the wastewater system through feces, urine, saliva, and other sources. Household wastewater is discharged into the sewer system and collected at the inflow to the wastewater treatment plant, where sampling occurs. The sample is then transported to a laboratory where it is analyzed, and the data are analyzed and published on internal- or external-facing dashboards. These data are then used by state, tribal, local, territorial, and national officials to support decision making on public health interventions, and the distribution of resources and support public communication.

SOURCE: Adapted from https://www.cdc.gov/healthywater/surveillance/pdf/Wastewater-COVID-infographic-h.pdf.

Current SARS-CoV-2 virus levels by site, United States

Current virus levels category	Num. sites	% sites	Category change in last 7 days
New Site	47	3	0%
0% to 19%	449	33	5%
20% to 39%	578	43	-5%
40% to 59%	216	16	-10%
60% to 79%	57	4	-12%
80% to 100%	7	1	0%

Total sites with current data: 1354

Total number of wastewater sampling sites: 1443

How is the current SARS-CoV-2 level compared to past levels calculated?

Select legend categories to filter points on the map.

New site ● 0% to 19% ● 20% to 39% ● 40% to 59% ● 60% to 79% ● 80% to 100% ● No recent data

New York City

DC

US Virgin Islands

Puerto Rico

Hawaii

Alaska

Guam

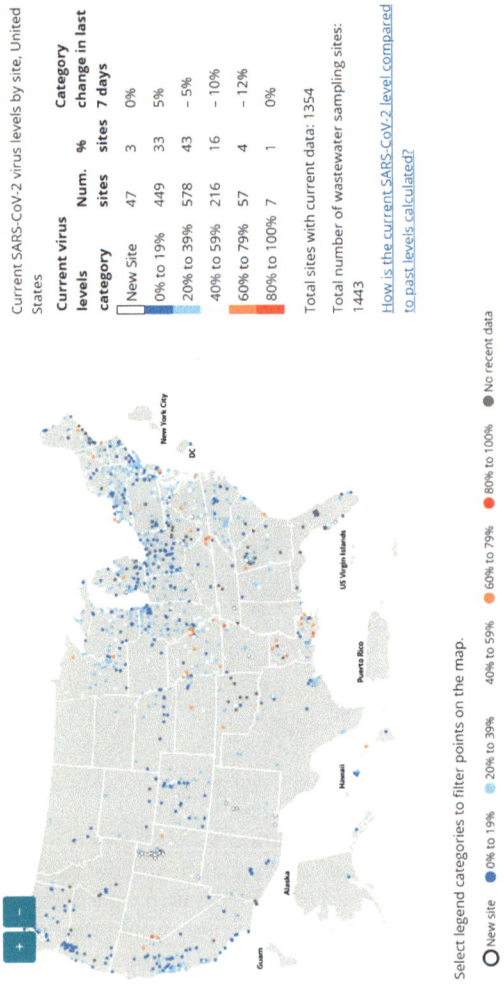

FIGURE 1-2 SARS-CoV-2 virus levels by site as of April 2024, as presented in the National Wastewater Surveillance System dashboard. The metric compares current SARS-CoV-2 levels with historical levels at the same site, with 0% indicating the lowest virus level and 100% indicating the highest virus level recorded at that site.
SOURCE: https://covid.cdc.gov/covid-data-tracker/#wastewater-surveillance.

wastewater treatment plant can range widely, from very small plants that serve as few as 100 people to large plants that serve a few million people, with a median of approximately 45,000 people (A. Kirby, CDC, personal communication, 2022).

Implementation of wastewater surveillance depends upon three primary entities—the local wastewater utility, analytical laboratory, and health department—to collect, test, and analyze samples and interpret the data (see Figure 1-1). Typically, local wastewater utilities collect, package, and ship the samples, which are used only for infectious disease surveillance and have no water quality regulatory implications. A public health, commercial, or academic laboratory partner analyzes the samples and reports the data to CDC and the local public health jurisdiction. The public health department interprets the data to identify trends regarding infection prevalence within a community, integrates the wastewater data with other surveillance data, determines the appropriate public health actions, and communicates this information to the general public. The public health department must agree to the data sharing policies of the CDC to participate (see Chapter 4). The multidisciplinary nature of a national wastewater surveillance system requires extensive collaboration between and across health departments, testing laboratories, and wastewater utilities. These partnerships and the demands on the participating entities are discussed further in the committee's Phase 1 report (NASEM, 2023).

CDC plays an important role to facilitate the overall function and operation of the NWSS as a national system and supports its continued development. In addition to providing ELC funding for local, state, and tribal wastewater surveillance (including staff time, sample collection, and analysis), CDC aggregates data from participating wastewater surveillance sites across the country that are submitted from public health jurisdictions and/or analytical laboratories. CDC then shares the results with the public, health officials, and policy makers through a variety of mechanisms, including a public-facing data dashboard, summarized data briefs, and a restricted-access data dashboard for health departments (Data Collation and Integration for Public Health Event Response [DCIPHER]). The goal of the NWSS is for these data to be interpreted by public health officials and used to inform community health interventions, raise public awareness of disease transmission within communities, and track pathogen dynamics across the nation. At a national scale, the information can inform decisions on allocations of federal resources and other support to states; at state, local, and tribal levels, the information can inform decisions on public health actions.

In support of the NWSS, CDC collaborates and coordinates with other federal agencies, such as the U.S. Environmental Protection Agency, U.S. Department of Homeland Security, and the National Institutes of Health, and coordinates communities of practice in conjunction with partners at the Water Environment Federation (WEF) and the Association of Public Health Laboratories (APHL). The communities of practice work to build capacity among the participating localities, host monthly meetings with cohorts of participants across jurisdictions to share experiences and keep health officials apprised of updates or program improvements, and facilitate connections among health departments that express a desire to share their data with one another. CDC also funds four NWSS Centers of Excellence—in California; Colorado; Houston, Texas; and Wisconsin—which provide additional expertise to assist with training, communication, and ongoing development of the NWSS. These Centers of Excellence complement an active research community that has helped facilitate the rapid evolution of wastewater epidemiology.

PHASE 1 REPORT

In late 2021, CDC charged the National Academies of Sciences, Engineering, and Medicine to appoint a committee of academic and public health experts to review community-level wastewater surveillance and its potential value toward understanding and preventing infectious disease in the United States. The committee's work was divided into two parts. The first phase, released in early 2023, provided an assessment of the usefulness of community-level wastewater surveillance in the United States and its potential value for infectious disease beyond COVID-19. (See Box 1-1 for the committee's complete Phase 1 statement of task.)

In its Phase 1 report (NASEM, 2023), the committee noted that wastewater surveillance has proved to be a valuable component of the nation's emergency response to the COVID-19 pandemic and will remain a critical data source for public health action in responding to COVID-19. Notably, as at-home testing increased and clinical laboratory testing and reporting decreased over the course of the pandemic, wastewater surveillance for new variants and their spread assumed increasing importance. The report stated that the pandemic spurred tremendous innovation and technological advances in wastewater surveillance, and ongoing knowledge development can help address gaps and improve analytical methods and data interpretation, not only for COVID-19 but also for newly emergent and re-emerging infectious diseases.

Based on the experience with wastewater surveillance during COVID-19, the report concluded that wastewater surveillance is worthy of further development and continued investment. The committee presented a vision for a national wastewater surveillance system that is flexible, equitable, sustainable, integrated, and actionable, and recommended approaches to address ethical and privacy concerns and develop a more representative wastewater surveillance system. In looking beyond COVID-19 toward additional microbial targets, the National Academies (NASEM, 2023) recommended three criteria to guide the NWSS in selecting among potential targets in its strategic allocation of effort and resources: (1) the public health significance of the threat, (2) the analytical feasibility for wastewater surveillance, and (3) the usefulness of community-level wastewater surveillance data to inform public health action. The report proposed a transparent process for prioritizing new targets and periodically re-evaluating their usefulness as scientific knowledge, technology, and infectious disease risks evolve.

The Phase 1 report emphasized the need for partnerships among federal agencies, nongovernmental organizations, academia, industry, wastewater utilities, and public health jurisdictions. The report highlighted the need to engage wastewater treatment plants as full partners to provide critical expertise and the value of close cooperation with researchers to further advance foundational knowledge needed for a robust surveillance system. The report also emphasized the importance of predictable and sustained federal funding moving forward (NASEM, 2023).

PHASE 2 STUDY AND CONTEXT

As the nation transitions from COVID-19 pandemic emergency response to endemic disease management with ongoing monitoring of emerging SARS-CoV-2 variants, the addition of new pathogen targets at some sites, and heightened awareness of potential pandemic risks, the application of wastewater surveillance as a public health tool also continues to evolve. In Phase 2 of the study (see Box 1-1), CDC asked the National Academies for a detailed assessment of opportunities and barriers in wastewater surveillance for the prevention and control of infectious diseases in the United States as it considers the future of the NWSS beyond COVID-19. CDC requested that the committee define specific characteristics for sampling, testing, and data analysis in the development of a robust, integrated national wastewater surveillance program and identify significant technical limitations and research and development needs. In its analysis, the committee considered approaches and methods used within NWSS, WastewaterSCAN, and other smaller programs where information was readily available. In this report, more attention was directed to NWSS, because it encompasses nearly all current community wastewater-based surveillance sites in the United States. Additionally, the NWSS is managed by the sponsor of this study. The committee focused on technical feasibility and scientific issues; although assessing the return on investment is also important, the question of the cost-effectiveness of wastewater surveillance in terms of the value of information provided is beyond the committee's charge.

To address its Phase 2 statement of task, the committee held six infor-mation-gathering meetings between April and October 2023. These discus-sions served as the initial basis for the committee's deliberations, which were further informed by a review of relevant literature and the committee's collective expertise. Knowing that wastewater surveillance was developed under emergency conditions and the science of wastewater epidemiology is rapidly evolving, the committee approached its task envisioning what should be accomplished in the next 5–8 years to increase the utility of wastewater surveillance in the United States at a national scale. Although many of the committee's recommendations can be acted upon sooner, the committee recognized that substantial research and development may

---

BOX 1-1
Statement of Task

Phase 1

An ad hoc committee of the National Academies of Sciences, Engineering, and Medicine will review community-level wastewater-based disease surveillance and its potential value toward prevention and control of infectious diseases in the United States. The committee will

1. Describe wastewater-based disease surveillance and how it differs from other approaches to disease surveillance and other wastewater monitoring for contaminants.
2. Review how wastewater-based surveillance has been useful in understanding COVID-19 in communities and informing local public health decisions.
3. Examine the potential value of specific applications of wastewater-based dis-ease surveillance for understanding and preventing disease and illness beyond COVID-19 and factors that may limit its application in the United States.
4. Describe the general characteristics of a robust, integrated approach for na-tional use of wastewater-based disease surveillance.
5. Discuss broad approaches to increase the public health impact of wastewater surveillance in the United States and the most effective strategies for federal, state, and local coordination to achieve national implementation of wastewater surveillance for an array of diverse infectious disease health indicators.

For the purpose of this study, community-level wastewater-based disease surveil-lance implies sampling at wastewater treatment plants and does not include local sur-veillance at neighborhood or institutional scales. To inform the study, the committee will briefly review ongoing and planned U.S. federal, state, local, tribal, and territorial efforts as well as international case examples for implementing wastewater-based disease surveillance. The committee's report will include conclusions and recommendations on wastewater-based surveillance in federal, state, and local public health efforts in the prevention and control of infectious diseases. Applications of wastewater-based

be needed to support decisions on the evolution of national wastewater surveillance.

The committee's vision and recommendations were developed assuming stable continued financial support for national wastewater surveillance and related research and development. In early conversations about the statement of task, CDC staff clarified that the intent of the task to "identify resources for supporting wastewater surveillance" was for the committee to recommend other partners or programs that could provide needed expertise, capabilities, and tools—not who should provide funding for the program. However, it is important to acknowledge the budget uncertainty for wastewater surveillance that lies ahead. Only late in the committee process did it

---

surveillance for noninfectious agents, in global settings, and for facility-level surveillance are outside the scope of this review, but the committee may identify these for future evaluation.

Phase 2

The committee will conduct an in-depth study of opportunities and barriers relevant to increasing the use and utility of wastewater surveillance for the prevention and control of infectious diseases in the United States. Specifically, the committee will

1. Define specific characteristics for development and implementation of a robust, integrated wastewater-based infectious disease surveillance program and discuss technical constraints and opportunities associated with wastewater sampling, testing, and data analysis, including
   - Methods and/or quality criteria, including genomics and sequencing, to detect pathogens, including strain- or variant-specific methods. Methods for discovery of unknown emerging pathogens can also be considered.
   - Data reporting, data analysis, and data interpretation for detecting emerging threats to public health and estimating disease incidence and prevalence, including data integration with other surveillance data for improving predictive models.
2. Identify significant technical limitations that could impact the feasibility of using wastewater surveillance as a platform for generating data for indicators of public health status and risk.
3. Describe the research, development, and information sharing needed to meet emerging needs and increase impact of wastewater surveillance for improving public health in the United States.
4. Identify resources for supporting wastewater surveillance.

In addition to its focus on community-level wastewater-based disease surveillance (i.e., with samples taken at a wastewater treatment plant), the committee may also discuss sub-sewershed sampling that would usefully support a robust, equitable, and sustainable wastewater surveillance program.

become evident that NWSS funding was facing sharp cuts. The President's Budget for FY 2025 (OMB, 2024) released in March 2024 included only $20 million for the NWSS, down from approximately $125 million/year during the pandemic, although local, state, and tribal programs can continue to use available funds previously allocated through ELC cooperative agreement grants for wastewater surveillance through FY 2027. The committee was not asked to restructure the NWSS under significantly reduced funding. Instead, the committee addressed its charge by laying out a vision toward a robust, integrated national wastewater-based infectious disease surveillance program with increased utility for the prevention and control of infectious diseases (see Box 1-1). As described in this report, achieving this vision and building a system that helps communities address endemic disease outbreaks while also ensuring a well-functioning wastewater surveillance system that is ready for the next pandemic will require much from CDC and substantial federal investment in research and analysis.

REPORT STRUCTURE

This report describes the state of wastewater surveillance sampling, testing, and data analysis and issues that should be addressed to improve the usefulness of data for public health response for a variety of pathogens and determinants of antimicrobial resistance. Chapters 2 through 5 focus on endemic pathogens, which are known to be present in the United States but may have regional, seasonal, or year-to-year variability in their prevalence, leading to outbreaks of concern to communities or the nation, while Chapter 6 addresses emerging pathogens and antimicrobial resistance of concern. Chapter 2 reviews trade-offs among sampling strategies. In Chapter 3, the committee evaluates the state of analytical methods and quality control and recommends areas for improvement. Chapter 4 reviews the tools available for data analysis, integration, and interpretation. Chapter 5 discusses the potential expansion of endemic targets for community-level wastewater surveillance. Finally, Chapter 6 addresses wastewater surveillance strategies (i.e., sampling, analytical methods, and data analysis and interpretation) for emerging outbreaks and pandemic threats, including those that are previously known outside the United States or in animal populations as well as truly unknown pathogens.

2

Sampling Methods for Endemic Pathogens

In this chapter, the committee discusses sampling approaches for a national wastewater surveillance system focused on endemic pathogens. Endemic pathogens are consistently present in the country but may have regional, seasonal, or year-to-year variability in their prevalence, leading to outbreaks of concern to communities or the nation. A system focused on endemic pathogens would require different sampling approaches than systems focused on emerging pathogen spread and outbreaks, which are discussed in Chapter 6. The committee provides an overview of the major considerations of the methods for wastewater sampling strategies, including spatial distribution, temporal distribution, and sampling methods. As discussed in the committee's Phase 1 report (NASEM, 2023), close collaboration with wastewater treatment plants, which provide samples and expertise, and dedicated resources to enable their participation are integral to any effort to improve sampling for wastewater surveillance.

OVERARCHING CONSIDERATIONS

Unlike clinical samples collected from a single person, wastewater samples represent a composite of the biological material of many individuals—from a few hundred to a few million. Available wastewater surveillance sampling strategies have different trade-offs in terms of the representativeness of the sample, equipment cost and maintenance, and staffing cost and capacity. Representativeness in wastewater surveillance can be described as how well the sample captures an equivalent amount of the pathogen biomarkers shed by infected individuals in the sewershed over a specified time period.

When considering wastewater sampling strategies for endemic pathogens, it is perhaps helpful to first envision an ideal or extreme sampling scenario that would provide the best possible representation of pathogen inputs from the community to better understand the trade-offs of sampling decisions.

An ideal wastewater sampling scenario for disease surveillance would involve every sewered community, with each sample including equivalent amounts of each person's fecal matter, urine, and other bodily secretions deposited throughout the previous 24-hour period in the sewershed. In this way, sample material (e.g., feces, urine) from a single infection in the community could be captured in every sample. In this scenario, "ideal" composite samples would be collected every day in every sewershed—or even sub-sewersheds for higher spatial resolution—in the country. Were this technically and financially feasible, the full dynamics of pathogen shedding in every sewered community could be captured. Even under this ideal scenario, interpretation may be challenged by natural variability, such as variation in shedding rates among infected individuals and wastewater flow rates. The other extreme may be where a small grab sample (a single sample taken at one point in time) is collected from a sewershed rarely, both temporarily and geographically. Where a sampling strategy should fall on the spectrum from grab samples collected rarely (e.g., monthly) in very limited locations to near-perfect 24-hour composite samples collected daily in every sewershed depends on the intended use of the information, wastewater treatment plant staff capacity for sampling, and funding constraints.

Much has been learned about the trade-offs in wastewater sampling to assess trends in COVID-19, but the potential addition of other targets beyond SARS-CoV-2 (see Chapter 5) necessitates consideration of their optimal sampling strategies and the costs and benefits of implementing a common sampling strategy for all. As the wastewater surveillance system evolves for other use cases or priorities, the optimal sampling frequency, sampling site distribution, and even sample volume to achieve actionable data on a specific target may vary.

SPATIAL DISTRIBUTION

In this section, the committee discusses the spatial distribution of NWSS sampling at state and national levels, including potential benefits of finer-scale sampling, such as sub-sewershed and facility sampling.

Spatial Distribution of NWSS Sampling Sites

Wastewater surveillance sites were brought into the National Wastewater Surveillance System (NWSS) during the public health crisis of the COVID-19 pandemic, and site selection was mainly driven by the ability of wastewater treatment plants to provide samples and the analytical capabilities of jurisdictions. In the committee's Phase 1 report (NASEM, 2023) the committee recommended a national wastewater surveillance system that is flexible, equitable, integrated, actionable, and sustainable. To achieve this vision, the committee recommended that the spatial distribution of sites be subject to intentional design, with adjustments as needed to optimize the network to address its intended purpose(s) without unnecessary redundancies to allow the system to be sustainable for decades to come. The NWSS sampling network should also be designed to be representative of the underlying population (NASEM, 2023). In additon to considering the overall coverage of the population, a representative sampling network for endemic pathogens should be

- Geographically representative, including socioeconomic and demographic differences in the U.S. population; and
- Able to capture key at-risk populations (e.g., communities with high social vulnerability or populations that are at higher risk for particular target pathogens).

Individual states and jurisdictions typically assess where surveillance should be done within their own unique constituencies based on their knowledge of at-risk communities. This necessitates a degree of flexibility in the structure of a national system to ensure it is at least partially customizable based on local needs.

As shown in Figure 2-1, current sampling sites are not evenly distributed across states, and tend to cluster in more populated, urban areas. Many rural counties, which are often disproportionately non-sewered, are not monitored. Roughly 14 percent of the U.S. population lives in a rural area (Dobis et al., 2021), and approximately 7 percent of NWSS sites are located in rural areas (i.e., urban-rural designation 6; see Figure 2-2). Although the residences in non-sewered locations are not directly sampled in wastewater surveillance systems, useful information can still be gained from neighboring communities if a subset of the population commutes to a sewered area for work, school, or other regular activities (e.g., errands, religious/social activities) (Figure 2-3; Yu et al., 2024). In terms of socioeconomic spatial patterns, NWSS sites appear to be relatively evenly spread across a range of levels of social vulnerability (see Figure 2-4).

Many jurisdictions are currently examining their spatial distribution of sampling to maximize the information for public health decision making with available resources, but very few optimization efforts have been completed. Research is under way in California using statistical tools to optimize the wastewater sampling network considering factors such as population served, population density, geographic coverage, Social Vulnerability

a)

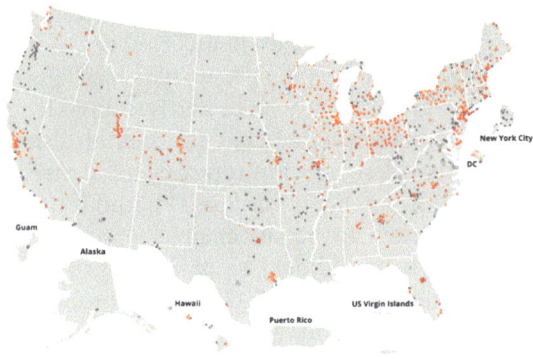

b)

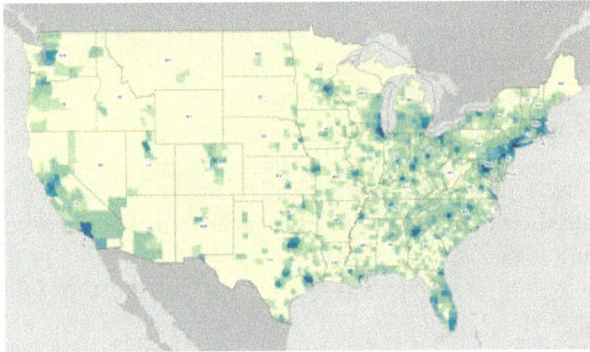

FIGURE 2-1 Spatial distribution of (a) NWSS as of January 2024, compared to demographic measures: (b) population density at the county level.
SOURCES: (a) https://covid.cdc.gov/covid-data-tracker/#wastewater-surveillance; (b) https://maps.geo.census.gov/ddmv/map.html.

Index, and the dissimilarity of wastewater surveillance signals (Daza-Torres et al., 2024). These tools can be used to evaluate the representativeness of their wastewater surveillance sampling network and whether vulnerable populations are adequately monitored. They can also be used to develop spatial sampling that provides a more comprehensive understanding of disease dynamics while minimizing redundancy. Redundancy can be assessed by evaluating differences among sites in historic data trends, signal magnitude, and timing, although redundancy is a pathogen-specific attribute. Under more drastic budget cuts, these statistical tools can be used to assess the relative value of information from existing sites, considering state or local priorities.

Bar Plot of Site Count per Urban-Rural Designation
Sites touching multiple counties counted in each.

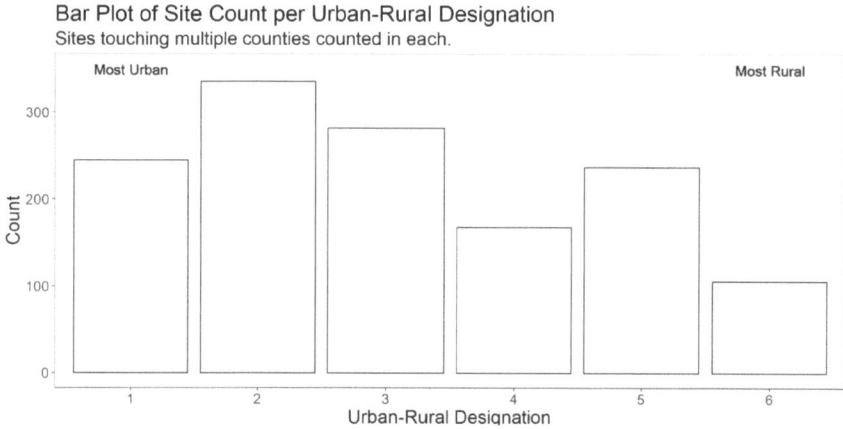

FIGURE 2-2 Histogram of sampling sites by urban-rural designation by county. The urban-rural designations (Ingram and Franco, 2013) include (1) counties with a large central population in a metropolitan statistical area (MSA) of 1 million or more (e.g., inner cities), (2) noncentral counties in MSAs of 1 million or more population (e.g., suburbs), (3) counties in MSAs of 250,000–999,999 people, (4) counties in MSAs of populations less than 250,000, (5) counties in micropolitan areas with between 10,000 and 50,000 people, and (6) noncore (or rural) counties, which lack an urban cluster of at least 10,000 people.
SOURCE: Committee, based on NWSS data found at data.cdc.gov.

It is important to note that different pathogens may exhibit different spatial and temporal transmission patterns; two sites that show similar wastewater surveillance results for SARS-CoV-2 in terms of the timing of peaks and trends may differ for another pathogen. Transmission route, transmissibility, and prevalence may all influence the spatiotemporal patterning (and degree to which two sites are redundant) in different ways across different pathogens. Therefore, optimization efforts will need to be revisited if new pathogen targets are added and potentially as pathogen variants evolve. The holistic national spatial representation will also need to be examined to ensure equity across the systems and that larger regional and national comparisons are possible.

Many state jurisdictions currently lack the capabilities to conduct these sampling optimization analyses. Given the potential for these analyses to improve the use of resources by reducing redundant sites and identifying critical gaps in coverage, the Centers of Disease Control and Prevention (CDC) should provide technical support for sampling optimization, including guidance for optimization rules of thumb and experts who can conduct the analyses in partnership with states. This is also an active area of research, and participation from the broader scientific and public health research community in developing optimization methods and optimal sampling strategies would benefit the NWSS.

16

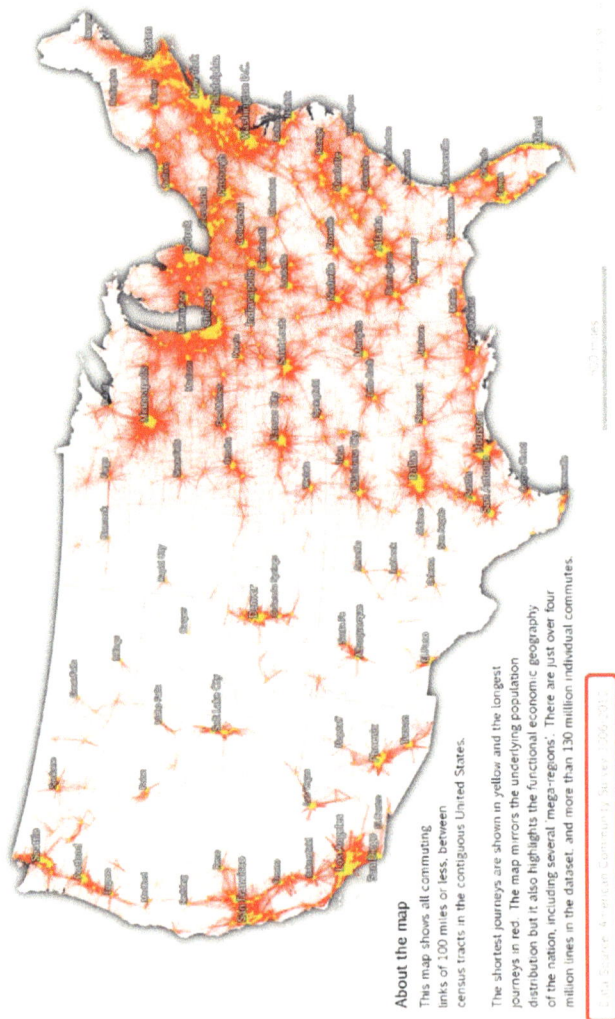

About the map

This map shows all commuting links of 100 miles or less, between census tracts in the contiguous United States.

The shortest journeys are shown in yellow and the longest journeys in red. The map mirrors the underlying population distribution but it also highlights the functional economic geography of the nation, including several mega-regions. There are just over four million lines in the dataset, and more than 130 million individual commutes.

FIGURE 2-3 Commuting networks for commutes ≤100 miles, from the U.S. Census Longitudinal Employer-Household Dynamics Origin-Destination Employment Statistics (LODES) data from 2006–2010. Many individuals in rural regions commute to urban centers for their regular work commute, with shorter commutes shown in yellow and longer commutes shown in red.
SOURCE: https://lehd.ces.census.gov/doc/workshop/2017/Presentations/TheaEvans.pdf.

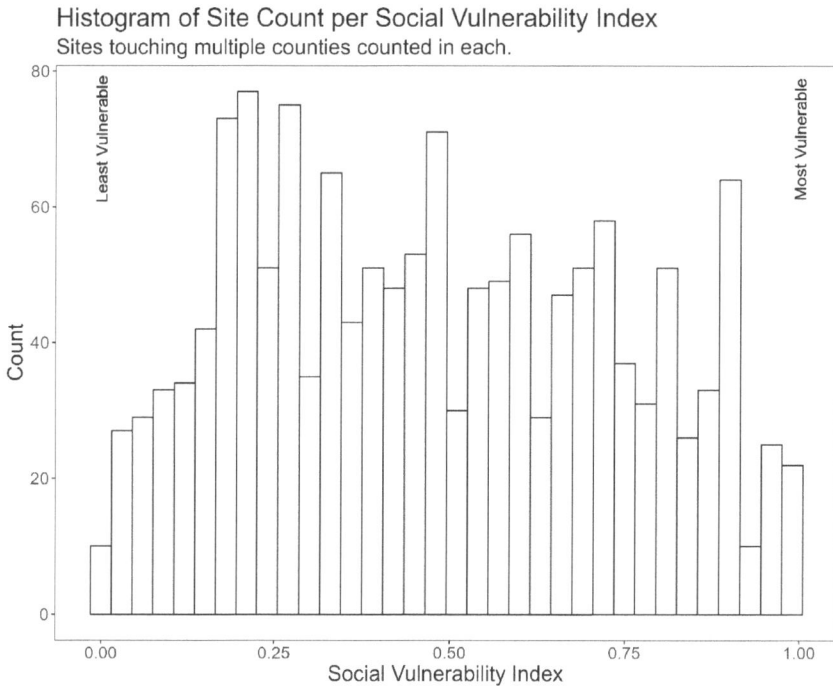

FIGURE 2-4 Histogram showing the number of NWSS sampling locations by Social Vulnerability Index (SVI) of the county where the site is located, with 1 as the most vulnerable (with social vulnerability defined as "the potential negative effects on communities caused by external stresses on human health") and 0 as the least vulnerable. Sites touching multiple counties are counted in each.
NOTE: For more information on the Centers for Disease Control and Prevention (CDC)/Agency for Toxic Substances and Disease Registry (ATSDR) SVI metric, see https://www.atsdr.cdc.gov/placeandhealth/svi/index.html.
SOURCE: Committee, based on NWSS data found at data.cdc.gov and CDC county-level national SVI designations.

The extent to which NWSS sites are representative of rural populations cannot be determined solely by geographic data (e.g., urban-rural indices), due to issues of mobility and contact between populations. Continued research would help states and CDC evaluate which rural and non-sewered areas more closely mirror sewered populations than others due to differences in population mixing. Further research on this issue using the Longitudinal Employer-Household Dynamics Origin-Destination Employment Statistics (LODES) data (see Figure 2-3), cell phone mobility data, and contact survey data (Dorélien et al., 2020; Mousa et al., 2021) would be highly beneficial in efforts to optimize the spatial distribution of sites and understand the extent to which non-sewered populations may be represented in existing sampling (e.g., via commuting for work or school). Additional research could evaluate whether or to what extent modeling and statistical tools can help adjust results from existing sites to better understand infectious disease trends in communities that are missing from the NWSS.

Consideration of Sampling Scale for Public Health Action

Although most NWSS sites provide community-level data by means of wastewater treatment plant sampling, there are advantages in facility or sub-sewershed sampling to address specific needs. It is important to understand that the reliability of the wastewater trend relative to an outbreak trend is impacted by the scale of the sewershed. Models of COVID outbreaks combined with individual fecal shedding dynamics highlight the impact of scale on wastewater signals (see Figure 2-5). In the simulated example provided in Figure 2-5, as a community's population decreases, the wastewater signals become more stochastic and are less likely to follow the COVID-19 prevalence in the community. This simulated scenario assumes complete mixing within the sewershed and no-sampling-induced variability (i.e., an ideal composite sample); neither of these is achievable in real systems. Thus, a real-world scenario would show even greater variability in smaller sewersheds. Trends observed from sewersheds, sub-sewersheds, and facilities containing small populations (e.g., <1000 individuals for SARS-CoV-2) may not accurately reflect illness trends in a community.

Sub-sewershed sampling. In cities with a single wastewater treatment plant representing a large population (e.g., over 1 million people), it can be more difficult to understand disease trends because increases in one part of the city could be offset by decreases in another, or an outbreak in a small neighborhood may be diluted by the rest of the sewershed. In such circumstances, higher-resolution sub-sewershed sampling (e.g., at manholes or lift stations within the sewershed) can be helpful for the purpose of verifying locations of concern. Sample collection within the sewershed reduces the represented population size to those more in line with small to mid-sized wastewater treatment plants. Additionally, sub-sewershed sampling may allow focused disease surveillance for specific localized at-risk groups, although the definition of who is at risk is likely to differ for different pathogens.

Sub-sewershed sampling is more complex than wastewater treatment plant sampling. A good understanding of the flow dynamics of the conveyance system is needed to choose sites and to understand the population represented by the sample. Flow rates are more variable in smaller areas of the system and therefore more challenging to measure but are necessary to understand loads and trends. Nonquantitative presence/absence measurements are typically easier to determine, but harder to interpret for trends.

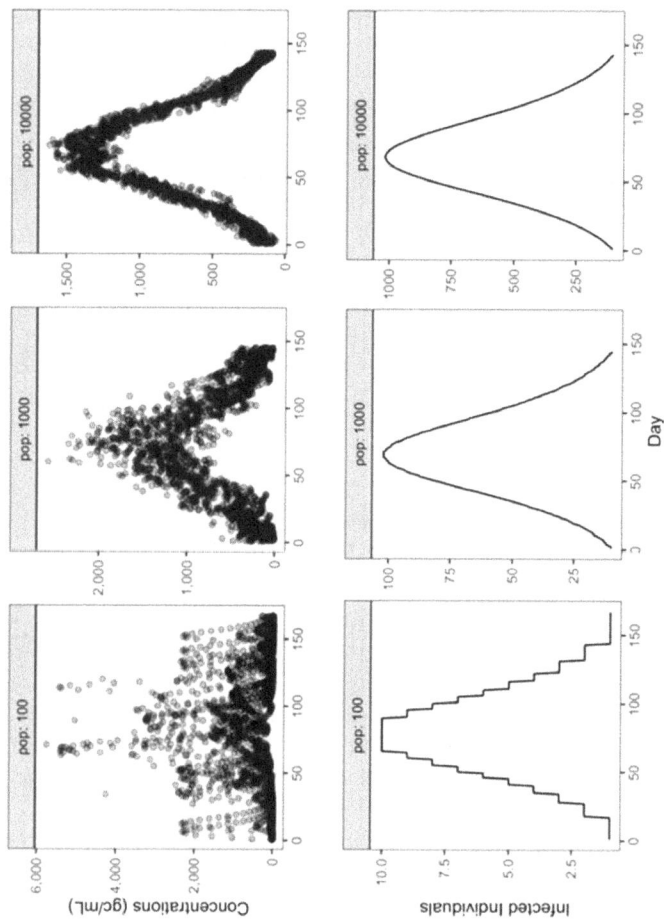

FIGURE 2-5 Predicted wastewater concentrations in ideally mixed and perfectly composited samples from sewersheds containing between 100 and 10,000 people (top row), relative to simulated outbreaks generated by Susceptible–Exposed–Infected–Recovered (SEIR) modeling (bottom row). Wastewater concentrations were generated from fecal shedding trajectories published in Arts et al. (2023).

SOURCE: Committee.

Further, sampling equipment may be vulnerable to vandalism if no secure location is available, and manhole access brings additional worker safety and traffic disruption issues, especially if located in high-traffic areas.

Facility-level sampling. Although monitoring individual facilities (e.g., nursing homes, prisons, hospitals, schools, universities, military bases) may not appear to be a high priority in a national wastewater surveillance system, facility-level surveillance has value to inform immediate interventions (e.g., resident screening, social distancing, hygiene protocols, educational outreach). This type of program can also provide a fine-scale picture of locations with the presence of target organisms, which provides an additional dimension to the understanding of disease spread at the community scale.

Facility-level sampling is particularly useful for understanding reservoirs of specific pathogens in the community or in subpopulations that have early incidence or higher disease risks than the general population, providing opportunities to mitigate outbreaks within these unique populations. For example, wastewater monitoring in hospitals, skilled nursing facilities, and assisted living facilities can help to understand the spread of rare antibiotic resistance targets and specific pathogens such as *Candida auris* due to the higher use of antibiotics and a more vulnerable patient and resident population in these facilities. Facility-level antimicrobial resistance surveillance would also be more actionable than wastewater treatment plant data because it is suspected to be less likely to be confounded by nonhuman or environmental reservoirs of resistance genes (Liu et al., 2023; McLellan and Roguet, 2019) but this has yet to be tested. A significant increase in wastewater detection of antibiotic-resistant genes at a facility could trigger investigation of whether there is an increased transmission and follow-up testing using appropriate clinical and clinical laboratory methods (see also Chapter 5).

Facility sampling can provide more actionable data, but states need to weigh these investments in sampling based on potential actions. By prioritizing monitoring and early detection at facilities with vulnerable populations (e.g., nursing homes, correctional facilities), wastewater surveillance can support highly impactful public health actions (see Box 2-1). However, jurisdictions should also weigh the complexity of interpretation and quality of the data at the facility level—the stochasticity and complications of measuring at small scales (due to variability in shedding, flow rates, etc., as shown in Figure 2-5) will be all the more challenging at the facility level. Particular issues arise in trying to obtain representative sampling at the facility level, because there is little mixing within such a small system and fecal shedding events pass through facilities so quickly. Sampling strategies for facilities are discussed later in this chapter. Also, some facilities may be more conducive than others for infectious disease surveillance. For example,

---

BOX 2-1
Wastewater Surveillance in Correctional Facilities

During the pandemic, wastewater surveillance was implemented in a number of correctional facilities to provide an early warning of a COVID-19 outbreak within the prison population to inform specific public health strategies to provide care and limit spread. Although collection and use of health data about incarcerated persons can raise special ethical concerns because of their vulnerability, wastewater surveillance also holds considerable promise for addressing health threats to this population. Correctional facilities represent high-risk groups for infectious disease transmission because of the densely housed population and typically poor ventilation. Outbreaks in prisons can easily spread to and from the community through prison staff and other prisons through prisoner transfers (Hassard et al., 2022).

Although wastewater can be challenging to sample at these sites because of limited access to prison wastewater infrastructure, researchers have identified statistically significant correlations between wastewater viral concentrations and clinical testing (Jobling et al., 2024; Klevens et al., 2023). A study of wastewater surveillance at a single large correctional facility in Georgia with 2,700 residents used passive sampling (Moore swabs) and reported that the polymerase chain reaction (PCR) signal was strongly correlated with clinical test results (Spaulding et al., 2023). The Ohio Department of Rehabilitation and Corrections conducted wastewater monitoring at 33 correctional facilities, with twice-weekly composite sampling (at least initially). Statistical tools were used to assess the trends through three or four sample moving averages and with machine learning tools. The wastewater surveillance data were useful to guide mitigation strategies, such as voluntary offender testing, staff testing, medical observation, controlling transport to a specific correctional facility during an outbreak, providing additional air-flow barriers, or determining whether to close gathering places, such as the commissary or barbershop (M. Weir, OSU, personal communication, 2023). As shown in Figure 2-5, it may be difficult for wastewater surveillance at small facilities to determine trends, and Hassard et al. (2022) noted that the minimum size of the population that can be usefully monitored for trends is unknown.

---

many K-12 students may not have bowel movements at school, which may reduce the representativeness of those data for fecally shed pathogens.

Selection of sampling scale. For typical endemic pathogens, wastewater treatment plant sampling will provide sufficient community-level data, but localities can evaluate the costs and benefits of additional sub-sewershed sampling. Facility- and subsewershed-level wastewater surveillance can provide valuable data to support early public health actions for vulnerable populations. Thus, use of NWSS funding for sub-sewershed and facility sampling may be appropriate if these data are sufficiently interpretable and can inform high-priority local, state, or national public health action related to the spread of infectious disease.

TEMPORAL DISTRIBUTION

Sampling frequency is an important consideration in all wastewater-based epidemiology applications. If sampling frequencies are too low, infections are missed, and trends are not observable. High-frequency sampling, however, is costly and may generate more information than is necessary for efficient public health action and may place a higher burden on wastewater treatment plants to provide these samples. There are several components of frequency that need to be considered when designing a surveillance program, including the frequencies with which samples are collected, shipped, and analyzed, as well as the frequency with which results are posted. For simplicity, the committee focused on how frequently samples are collected—assuming that shipment, analysis, and reporting would follow immediately—but implications of these other aspects of frequency are also discussed, and timeliness of reporting is addressed in Chapter 4. Because this chapter covers endemic pathogen monitoring, this discussion is focused on the frequency necessary to accurately detect trends as opposed to accurately detecting the presence or absence of a target. This is also applicable to monitoring infectious disease trends during local outbreaks. Temporal sampling considerations for presence/absence applications, such as monitoring for emerging pandemic threats at a large international event, are discussed in Chapter 6.

Most studies that have examined the frequency of samples necessary for correctly identifying trends have largely focused on SARS-CoV-2. Early studies correlated wastewater and case data retrospectively to identify the number of samples necessary to correctly observe trends (as defined by clinical cases). Studies demonstrated correlations in retrospective analysis with samples collected at a frequency as low as once per week (Duvallet et al., 2022). Feng et al. (2021) used Monte Carlo simulations to evaluate the impacts of sampling frequencies to identify a trend over a 3-week period and determined at least two samples per week were necessary to determine trends. Likewise, Graham et al. (2020) determined that sampling primary sludge twice per week was necessary for obtaining significant associations between case counts and wastewater concentrations. Based on these and other early findings, many surveillance programs selected twice-weekly sampling. For example, Ohio conducted SARS-CoV-2 monitoring two times per week (Feng et al., 2021).

More recent studies with larger data sets have highlighted the value of more frequent sampling for timely trend detection of SARS-CoV-2. Holst et al. (2022) compared SARS-CoV-2 data collected one or two times per week with data collected three to five times per week and determined that higher-frequency sampling provided more timely identification of outbreak onset and the higher resolution of trends. Schoen et al. (2022) determined that a sampling frequency of four times per week or greater was necessary to reduce the error associated with predicting incidence rates. Chan et al. (2023) tested for trends of SARS-CoV-2 wastewater measurements and found that sampling four or five times per week was necessary to effectively detect trends with a sensitivity and specificity cutoff of 0.5. These more recent studies demonstrate the potential value of higher-resolution sampling for the timely detection of trends with endemic pathogen surveillance.

One issue with many analyses focused on identifying the sampling frequency necessary to obtain trends is that trends are typically identified with a rolling average of multiple samples. These rolling average windows can quickly become too wide for timely decisions. For example, when samples are collected twice per week, a three-sample average captures samples from the previous 2 weeks of wastewater data to determine a trend (assuming a 4-day turnaround time). Increasing the number of samples in the rolling average analysis (e.g., using a five-sample rolling average) and continuing to sample twice per week may decrease noise in the detected trend; however, in this case the sampling window covers 3 weeks, which may be too wide of a window to capture timely shifts in trends when evaluating them in real time for public health decision making. A rolling window of 5–7 samples collected during the previous 1–2 weeks would substantially reduce the noise in the trend prediction and allow rapid response to changing trends in the community. Unfortunately, this will be too cost prohibitive for many programs and could exceed the staff capacity of some wastewater treatment plants. The trade-offs of sample frequency and rolling averages will need to be considered for each program. Based on the current state of the knowledge, the committee recommends that, during times when timely pathogen target trends from wastewater are critical (e.g., when a new variant is circulating or there is concern over a potential outbreak), sampling frequency of more than twice per week will be most valuable. Outside of these periods, when trends over many weeks are desired, sampling at once or twice per week may be acceptable. One possible approach to reduce the burden and cost while collecting higher-frequency samples is to batch the shipment and analyses of the samples. For example, samples could be collected at the plant on a daily or every-other-day basis but sent and analyzed only once or twice a week. This results in a high-frequency data set but saves time and costs for packaging, shipping, and possibly analysis, so long as the samples can be rapidly processed and reported once they do arrive.

Frequency recommendations will be dependent on the pathogen and overall goal of the sampling effort. To date, wastewater surveillance of endemic pathogens has generally focused on assessing pathogen trends. For reference, CDC currently recommends that at least one sample per week be collected for SARS-CoV-2 and that three measurements are necessary for a trend. The impact of sampling frequencies for determining trends of other pathogens has been much less studied. They could be different from SARS-CoV-2 due to differences in shedding levels and dynamics through the course of an outbreak. It may be most efficient to sample all targets on the same cadence due to economies of scale in laboratory and personnel costs, and SARS-CoV-2 will likely drive the frequency initially. For respiratory viruses, the committee estimates that twice-weekly sampling will be sufficient to determine trends, although data on sampling frequencies to support trend analysis of influenza and respiratory syncytial virus (RSV) are lacking. Many of the endemic pathogens of interest for wastewater surveillance have consistent seasonal trends. Influenza A and RSV cases, for example, tend to peak in the United States in winter and have few, if any, cases in summer months. Sampling and analysis for these targets could therefore decrease or pause during times when there is historically little illness activity and resume in time to detect early seasonal activity.

As mentioned above, in this section the committee has assumed that there is no delay between sample collection and sample reporting. The longer it takes for sample results to be reported, the longer the rolling average window and thus the older the detected trend. Currently, there are a range of workflow approaches, with substantial lag times between sample collection and data availability for some sites. Improvement is needed in all steps of the process to streamline the workflow and optimize data availability and relevance (see also Chapter 4).

In summary, the selection of a temporal sampling program will depend on the pathogen and the use case, which determines how rapidly trends need to be detected. Sampling at least two times per week for SARS-CoV-2, influenza, and RSV will generally lead to positive correlations between wastewater levels and cases and sufficiently timely determination of trends. Programs wishing to increase sampling frequency could consider batching the shipment and analysis of samples (e.g., 4 days of samples shipped and analyzed twice per week).

SAMPLING METHODS

There are multiple methods for collecting wastewater samples that are analyzed for endemic pathogens. Some of the considerations include the physical location of sample collection, whether the sampling is conducted manually or by an automated device, and what kind of wastewater sample is collected (e.g., solids or liquids). Trade-offs in the selection of sampling method include the correlation of the results with epidemiological data, the sensitivity and variability of the resulting data (i.e., if one approach is more amenable to lower detection limits or consistent data), the comparability of data across sampling sites, the representativeness of the samples for the population being monitored (and the ability to assess the representativeness of the samples), and the effort and cost of collecting, transporting, and processing the samples for analysis. At the time of this report, large wastewater surveillance programs in the United States use a variety of the methods. Biobot Analytics has focused primarily on 24-hour flow- or time-proportional composite influent samples collected from wastewater treatment plants or pump stations. The Michigan Wastewater Surveillance Network focuses on liquid wastewater samples collected, and the collection process varies across the network, with some groups focusing on grab samples and other groups focusing on flow- and time-proportional composite samples. Wastewater surveillance conducted by WastewaterSCAN,[1] with over 180 sampling sites across the United States, focuses on enriched solids samples, collected either in primary sedimentation basins at wastewater treatment plants or via manual sedimentation of influent.

In practice, most ongoing wastewater surveillance programs use the sampling method they selected early in the COVID-19 pandemic. This is due to many reasons, including the desire to have consistent data, the capital costs and training that went into their sampling program, and the preference for and trust in familiar methods. However, the transition of wastewater surveillance from a pandemic emergency response to a long-term national network designed to assist the prevention and control of infectious diseases necessitates that these trade-offs be reconsidered across a larger set of targets and broader intended uses of the data. In the following sections, the committee reviews the major approaches to wastewater sampling and the trade-offs that come with specific approaches.

Wastewater Treatment Plant Sampling Methods

Several different sampling methods can be used to collect samples at wastewater treatment plants (termed community-level wastewater surveillance). The most common methods include composite wastewater influent sampling, grab influent sampling, and the collection of primary sludge from treatment plant clarifiers (Figure 2-6). Representativeness is the most important consideration for sample collection at wastewater treatment plants because samples that are not representative can lead to sampling-derived variability in the resulting data. This in turn has a negative impact on the interpretation of the observed infectious disease trends and thus reduces the value of the data. Nonrepresentative results can lead to misinterpretation, inappropriate public health actions (either too much or too little action) in

---

[1] See https://www.wastewaterscan.org/en.

26

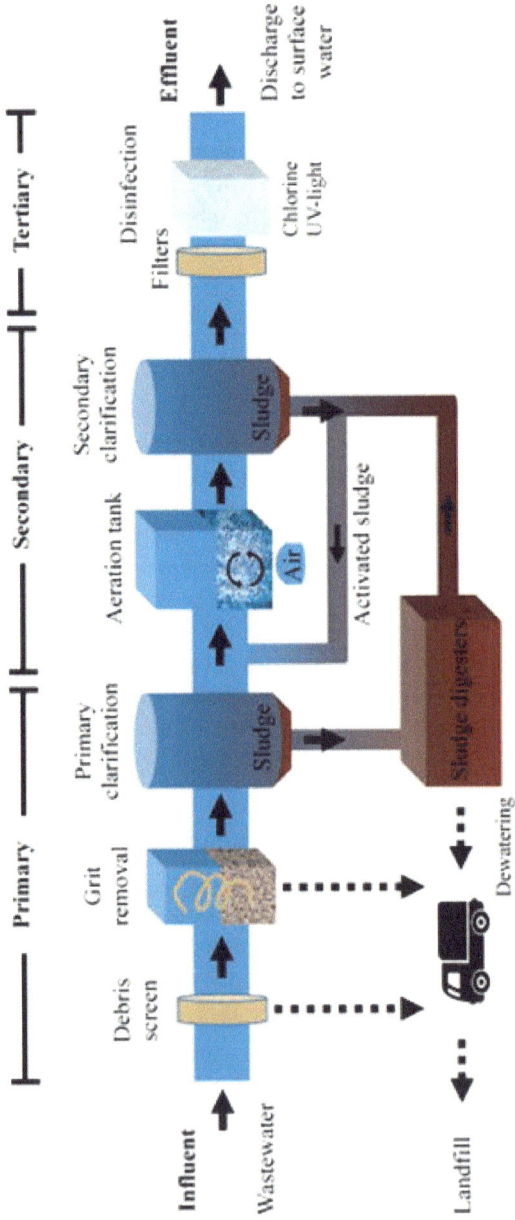

FIGURE 2-6 Wastewater treatment plant treatment processes.
SOURCE: Martin-Pozo et al., 2022.

response to the surveillance data, wasted resources, as well as eroded confidence in the data. The following provides a brief overview of these main sampling strategies and then discusses considerations and trade-offs with the different approaches.

Influent sampling from wastewater treatment plants entails collection of wastewater from the head of the wastewater treatment plant (i.e., where the influent enters), although there is some variability in sampling locations (e.g., true raw influent, after the screens or grit removal). Composite sampling occurs at regular intervals over a period of time (typically 24 hours), combining the individual samples into a composite sample (see Figure 2-7). In doing so, composite sampling captures a larger fraction of the material shed over the period of a day than would be captured with a single sample collected at a single point in time. The collection of composite samples can be conducted manually by collecting samples by hand from the influent flow at regular intervals and combining them into a composite sample or with equipment that automatically collects samples (i.e., autosamplers) from the wastewater treatment plant influent at regular intervals and combines the samples into a composite sample.

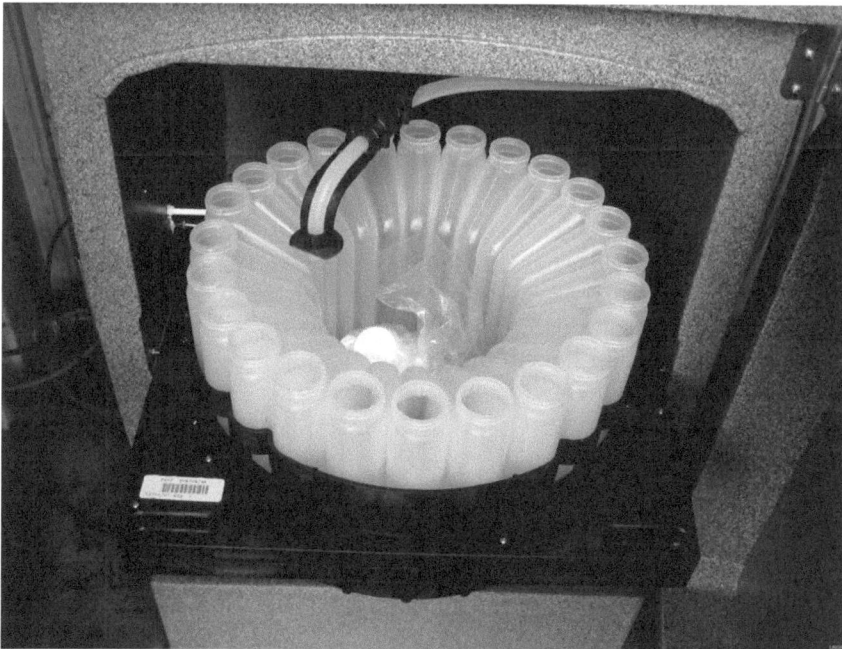

FIGURE 2-7 Composite sampling.
SOURCE: USGS, 2008. https://www.usgs.gov/media/images/automated-sampler

Composite Influent Sampling

There are different types of autosampling approaches, such as flow-weighted sampling, time-weighted sampling, and continuous composite sampling. Time-weighted composite sampling involves the collection of a certain volume of water for a specified duration over specified intervals. For example, a composite sampler may collect 100 mL of wastewater over a 5-minute period every hour. In this scenario, a total of 2.4 L would be collected over a 24-hour period. It is worth noting that in this case, the composite sample is only collected for about 8.3 percent of the 24-hour period. For the remaining 91.7 percent of the time, the wastewater is not being sampled. In flow-weighted sampling, the collected sample volume is proportional to the flow rate of the wastewater. For example, the sampler may collect 100 mL for every 100,000 L that flows into the wastewater treatment plant. In general, flow-weighted sampling is considered to be more representative than time-weighted sampling because it better captures the pathogen loads over time despite flow variability. This is because more sample is collected when more material is entering the wastewater treatment plant. Flow-weighted sampling requires accurate flow metering, which can sometimes be challenging to maintain.

Influent Grab Sampling

Grab sampling involves the manual collection of a water sample at one point in time. For the purpose of this discussion, grab sampling is defined here as the collection of a single grab sample, as opposed to the collection of multiple grab samples. (The latter would be referred to as composite sampling.) Grab samples are commonly collected by lowering a clean sample bottle into the wastewater flow (Figure 2-8). These samples are also generally collected at the head of the wastewater treatment plant, depending on accessible locations to the influent. Whereas the composite sample represents several snapshots in time, the grab sample is only representative of a single point in time.

Primary Sludge Sampling

In addition to samples collected from the head of wastewater treatment plants, enriched solids samples are sometimes collected from primary clarifiers at wastewater treatment plants (Figures 2-6 and 2-9). The purpose of this is to leverage the pathogen concentration process that inherently takes place at most wastewater treatment plants. Suspended solids in municipal wastewater are commonly settled from the bulk wastewater during primary

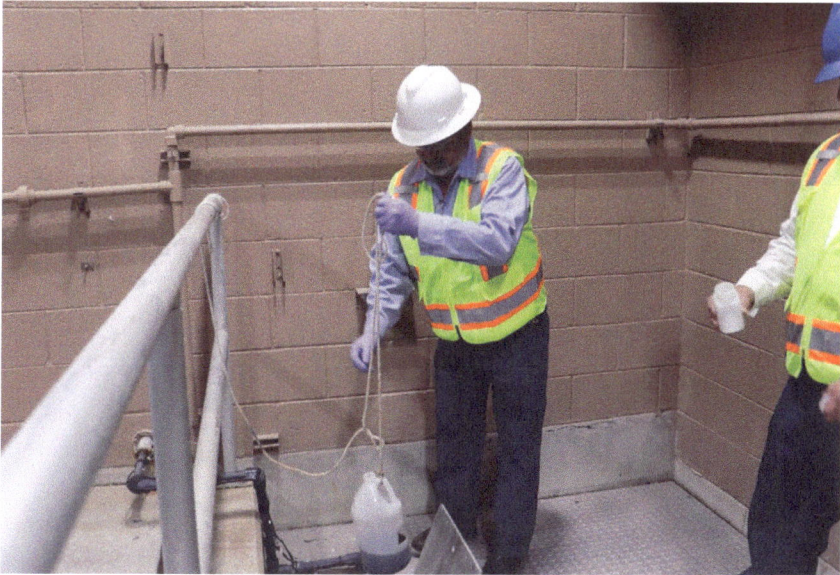

FIGURE 2-8 Grab sampling as part of wastewater surveillance at the Haskell R. Street Wastewater Treatment Plant in El Paso.
SOURCE: https://elpasomatters.org/2022/04/18/how-el-paso-is-using-wastewater-surveillance-to-detect-covid-19-spread/.

wastewater treatment. In this process, the wastewater spends time (typically ~2 hours) in a large basin and solids settle by gravity. Whereas the clarified wastewater passes to the next step of the wastewater purification process, the wastewater solids are collected from the underflow of sedimentation basins and these solids (termed primary sludge) are removed (via pipe flow) for further treatment and disposal. Suspended solids concentrations collected in primary sludge samples are typically in the range of 2 to 7 percent. This is in contrast to a concentration of <0.1 percent by mass in wastewater influent. Primary sludge samples are commonly captured from streams that are regularly pulled from the primary clarifiers. Some smaller plants do not have primary clarifiers; in these cases, influent samples are sometimes collected and settled manually to capture settled solids similar to what would be collected from primary clarifiers. The collected and transported solids can be further concentrated in the laboratory, often through centrifugation. Pathogens are then extracted from the enriched solids samples and quantified using methods similar to those used with influent sample concentrates.

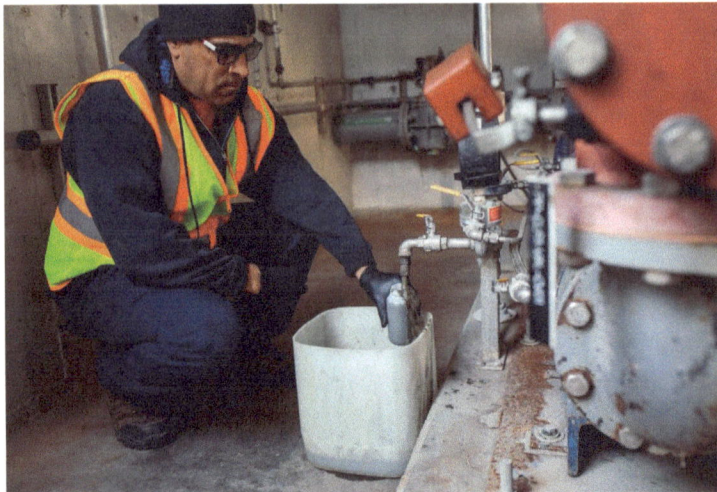

FIGURE 2-9 A utilities plant operator siphons wastewater sludge to be analyzed for evidence of SARS-CoV-2.
SOURCE: Anna Maria Barry-Jester/KFF Health News.

Considerations Affecting Grab Versus Composite Sampling

Single grab samples represent a snapshot at a fixed point in time, and the interpretation is limited by the potentially small fraction of the sewershed population captured in the sample. Composite samples, on the other hand, represent the average of a number of snapshots collected over a period of time and therefore usually result in measurements that are more representative of the sewershed population. Due to their better representativeness, composite influent samples are preferred for measuring trends in endemic pathogens. That being said, a composite sampling apparatus can cost in the range of $2,000 to $7,000 (Liu et al., 2022) or more, depending on the options, and requires more maintenance than single grab samples. Likewise, collecting multiple grab samples manually and combining them requires more labor and supplies than collecting a single grab sample. Consequently, the collection of composite samples is not always a feasible option due to staff or resource issues.

Results obtained with single grab samples can in some cases be reflective of composite samples. For example, similar results have been observed for paired grab and composite samples when the monitoring was focused on target presence versus absence (George et al., 2022; Kmush et al., 2022). For endemic pathogen surveillance, wastewater samples are more often analyzed for pathogen concentration trends rather than absence or presence. For this purpose, grab samples are more likely to result in concentrations similar to composite samples when collected from larger sewersheds (George et al., 2022; Kmush et al., 2022). For example, George et al. (2022) reported that SARS-CoV-2 RNA concentrations determined in grab samples were within 50 percent of concentrations of composite samples in a sewershed with approximately 50,000 inhabitants. By contrast, concentrations obtained with grab samples were up to two orders of magnitude different than composite samples in a sewershed representing 400 people. Curtis et al. (2020) also observed good correlations between grab and composite wastewater samples collected at the influent of a treatment plant representing a population of 78,000. In this case, 55 percent of the grab sample concentrations were within 50 percent of the concentrations obtained with composite samples. It is worth noting that these studies were conducted for SARS-CoV-2 at specific prevalence rates in the community—these relationships will differ with different pathogens and with different COVID-19 incidence.

The reason for these differences in how well single grab sample results reflect those obtained with composite samples is related to how human inputs vary and how flows vary between systems. The wastewater entering the treatment plant from larger systems exhibits less variability, both in flow and in constituent concentrations (e.g., total suspended solids concentration; see Table 2-1; Metcalf & Eddy et al., 2013). This is in part due to the larger number of contributors in larger wastewater samples—more inputs over time reduce the temporal variability observed within the sewer system.

TABLE 2-1 Ranges of Geometric Standard Deviations for Flow Rates and Common Wastewater Constituents in Typical Small (1–10 Mgal/day), Medium (10–100 Mgal/day), and Large (>100 Mgal/day) Wastewater Treatment Plants

	Ranges of Geometric Standard Deviations		
	Small Plants	Medium Plants	Large Plants
Flowrate	1.4–2.0	1.1–1.5	1.1–1.2
Total suspended solids (TSS)	1.4–2.1	1.3–1.6	1.1–1.3
Biochemical oxygen demand (BOD)	1.4–2.1	1.3–1.6	1.1–1.3
Chemical oxygen demand (COD)	1.5–2.2	1.4–1.8	1.1–1.5

NOTE: These data exclude systems with large amounts of infiltration into the collection system. Geometric standard deviation (GSD) is a measure of spread or variability in a quantity. For log-normally distributed quantities, it is expected that approximately 95% of the observations will be in a range between the geometric mean divided by the square of the GSD and the geometric mean multiplied by the square of the GSD.
SOURCE: Adapted from Metcalf & Eddy et al., 2013.

This is also in part due to the mixing characteristics in different conveyance systems. The extent to which the wastewater entering the treatment plant has mixed depends on factors such as the flow rate as well as how long different samples spend in the sewer, the physical aspects of the system (e.g. slope), and pumping that takes place in the system.

In summary, composite samples are, by nature, more representative than grab samples, and thus they are more reliable for assessing the overall occurrence of target organisms in a sewershed and provide more consistent and reliable data. Single grab samples cost the same to analyze as composite samples but the value of the data to understand trends is much lower, given the data variability. Therefore, composite sampling will typically be worth the additional investment costs. Single grab samples can be useful for assessing the presence or absence of a target, but negative results need to be weighed against the probability of detecting a signal. In large sewersheds, concentration trends obtained with single grab samples collected consistently at peak flow may be reflective of what would be captured with a composite sample, but ideally this should be validated against composite sampling during a period of time in which the pathogen target is present or changing (i.e., over 1–2 months), so that the degree of representativeness of grab samples is established. Grab samples collected in small sewersheds will likely have large variations associated with their measurements and this will decrease the reliability of their trend detection.

Considerations of Samples Enriched with Solids

As mentioned above, most wastewater surveillance studies and programs have focused on quantifying pathogens in wastewater treatment plant influent samples. Some programs keep the solid fraction in the wastewater sample prior to concentrating and extracting the target pathogens while others remove the solids prior to concentrating and extracting. However, several surveillance programs have focused on the collection and analysis on the solid fraction. Wastewater samples that are concentrated with solids are typically collected by sampling either the primary sludge (see Figures 2-6 and 2-9) or the wastewater influent and concentrating the solid fraction via settling, filtration, or centrifugation (Kim et al., 2022). Sample processing and analysis then focuses only on the concentrated solids fraction. Prior to discussing the benefits and drawbacks of focusing on samples enriched with solids, it is important to first understand the reasons pathogens are enriched in samples that contain more wastewater solids.

Municipal wastewaters contain suspended solids (i.e., particles > 0.2 µm), including solids of fecal origin. The wastewater that reaches the wastewater treatment plant is primarily liquid, with a total suspended solids content of <0.1 percent. As wastewater is conveyed to the wastewater treatment plant, the fecal samples are broken into smaller pieces, and pathogens that enter the wastewater from humans in feces, urine, saliva, and skin will partition between the solid and liquid phases until equilibrium is reached. Virus, bacteria, and protozoa particles exhibit a range of sorption or partition tendencies at equilibrium. These tendencies are frequently characterized by partition coefficients (K_d), which represent the ratio of the pathogen particle concentration in the solids to the concentration in the liquid. Reported K_d values for viral genomes in untreated wastewater are in the range of approximately 100 to 10,000 mL/g (Boehm et al., 2024). Note that the K_d values reported in the literature sometimes represent the partitioning of the infectious pathogen particles and other times represent the partitioning of the measured pathogens genes, which for viruses could include intact particles, damaged particles, and free nucleic acids. The reported K_d values for viruses suggest that at equilibrium, 1 g of dried wastewater solids contains the same number of viruses as between 100 mL and 10 L of wastewater liquids, depending on the virus being tested.

If at equilibrium, the fraction of pathogens in each phase of a specific wastewater sample depends on both the K_d of the pathogen and the percentage of solids in that wastewater sample (Table 2-2). Equilibrium between the liquid and solid fractions of wastewater may not be fully achieved in a sample, but partition coefficients provide an approach to predicting the relative pathogen concentrations in the wastewater liquids and solids. Assuming a pathogen has a K_d equal to 1,000 mL/g, a composite wastewater sample contains 0.1 percent solids (by dry weight), and the system is at equilibrium, 9 percent of the pathogens in a wastewater sample would be associated with the solid fraction of wastewater and 91 percent of

TABLE 2-2 Examples of Pathogen Partitioning at Equilibrium Between Wastewater Solids and Liquid at Equilibrium Based on Different Partition Coefficients and Total Suspended Solids Concentrations

Pathogen Partition Coefficient, K_d (mL/g)	Wastewater Total Suspended Solids Concentration (TSS, mg/L)	Percentage of Pathogens Partitioned to Solids in Wastewater
100	100	1%
1000	100	9%
1000	200	17%
1000	300	23%
10,000	100	97%

NOTE: These percentages were calculated as follows: .
SOURCE: Committee.

the pathogens would be associated with the liquid fraction. Research groups that focus on samples enriched with solids are harnessing this affinity of the viruses to wastewater solids. Indeed, a major advantage of collecting primary sludge is that it requires only a small sample volume (approximately 50 mL) to be collected and transported.

Pathogen concentrations measured in wastewater samples are commonly compared to clinical data to establish if the sampling method works. Nucleic acid concentrations obtained with both influent samples and primary sludge samples have correlated strongly with clinical cases for a number of pathogens. For example, Boehm et al. (2023a) found positive correlations for SARS-CoV-2, influenza A, influenza B, RSV A, RSV B, human metapneumovirus, rhinovirus, and seasonal coronaviruses when comparing the concentrations of RNA in primary sludge with positivity rates from clinical samples submitted to sentinel laboratories. Similar findings were reported for human norovirus (Boehm et al., 2023c) and enterovirus D68 (Boehm et al., 2023d) in primary sludge samples. Likewise, strong correlations between clinical cases and wastewater levels have been demonstrated with influent samples for a number of pathogens, including SARS-CoV-2 (Medema et al., 2020), human norovirus (Ammerman et al., 2024), and influenza A virus (Zheng et al., 2023). Overall, there is strong evidence that samples focused primarily on the liquid fraction (i.e., influent samples) and solids fractions (i.e., primary sludge samples) of wastewater can provide pathogen signals that are helpful for tracking disease trends in communities.

With respect to sensitivity and the ability to detect pathogens when community prevalence is low, limited studies have compared paired influent and primary sludge samples collected on the same day at times when prevalence is low. Some studies with paired influent and primary sludge samples have found that targeting the primary sludge, or more generally enriched solids samples, results in more positive detections (Graham et al., 2020; Wolfe et al., 2022), whereas others have reported similar sensitivities for paired liquid and enriched solids samples (Hewitt et al., 2022; Kim et al., 2022). These conflicting findings are likely due to the wide range of methods used in the studies and the different effective volumes and masses captured in the analyses. Furthermore, pathogens exhibit a range of partition coefficients, and so the relative sensitivity of influent versus primary sludge will differ from target to target. Finally, wastewater samples can contain high levels of inhibitors, and there may be differences in inhibition between sample types and methods (see Chapter 3). At this time, there is not sufficient evidence to determine if primary sludge or influent samples are overwhelmingly more sensitive.

Methods focused on influent or primary sludge should be similarly representative if the samples are both composite. The age of primary sludge samples collected from primary clarifiers is often reported by wastewater treatment plants. However, characterizing the specific age of solid samples collected under the primary clarifier is complicated, dynamic, and not something that is frequently measured by wastewater treatment plants. The age of the solids (or residence time) in the clarifier blanket can be estimated using the total suspended solids (TSS) concentrations in the clarifier influent and effluent along with the TSS mass in the clarifier sludge blanket, but primary clarifier sludge age is not often calculated by wastewater treatment plants. Furthermore, the mixing state of primary solids is highly dependent on the physical design of the sedimentation tank and on overall plant hydraulics. Without additional analysis of plant configurations and settling times, the representativeness of solid samples collected from sedimentation basins is less certain than solids from well-defined influent liquid composite sampling. Collecting an influent composite sample and manually settling the solids to concentrate pathogens can help define the composition of an enriched solids sample. In this case, the composition of the sample is easily defined (e.g., the sample represents solids enriched from a 24-hour flow-weighted composite sample).

Recommended Sampling Methods at Wastewater Treatment Plants

For wastewater surveillance where the collection point is at the wastewater treatment plant and the sample is influent, composite sampling is preferable because it is more likely to provide a representative sample of the sewershed. For small wastewater treatment plants (e.g., defined by the U.S. Environmental Protection Agency as serving <10,000), it is particularly important to use composite sampling to obtain a representative sample of the community, because the wastewater samples are likely to be more highly variable due to the variable shedding dynamics of infected individuals (see Table 2-1). Small communities may have fewer resources to support in-house expertise or equipment to perform composite sampling and may benefit from use of a contractor to deploy and maintain the autosampler if NWSS or state funding support is available. If a composite sampler is not feasible, multiple grab samples could be taken several hours apart and then combined to mimic a composite sample, although such an approach would require more time from wastewater treatment plant staff.

Primary sludge sampling has proven a sensitive and effective approach and has the advantage of small sample size. However, more work should be devoted to characterizing the retention time of the primary sludge at different sizes and configurations of wastewater treatment plants to determine what timescale of composite the sludge sample represents. More analysis of existing wastewater data is necessary to determine if analytical methods are more sensitive for detecting trends of endemic pathogens in common primary sludge samples compared to typical composite samples of wastewater influent. Furthermore, more research is needed to determine if pathogen data from primary sludge samples or influent samples are more directly comparable between different sewersheds. Ultimately, use of the same representative sampling methods across all sites would improve comparability across sites. However, more analysis is needed to examine the advantages and disadvantages of primary sludge versus influent samples before determining an optimal method for consistency, or at minimum different but comparable methods.

Sub-sewershed and Facility Sampling Methods

Several factors affect the sampling strategy appropriate for sub-sewersheds (frequently conducted via manholes), including the capacity for composite sampler placement, the sub-sewershed size, expected wastewater mixing, and the intended use of the data for targeted interventions (e.g., if quantitative data are necessary or if presence/absence data are sufficient). An effective grab sampling program will require more samples than composite sampling, and this may offset the cost of the composite sampling equipment. The likelihood of erroneous results increases with grab samples as the incidence of the target organisms decreases (George et al., 2022); in this case, negative results could produce a false sense of security. If monitoring is occurring for a targeted intervention that is effort or resource intensive, composite sampling may be worth the investment to get more reliable, quantitative results. The Houston Wastewater Epidemiology project, which is a CDC National Wastewater Surveillance System Center of Excellence, collects 24-hour time-proportional samples from its lift stations and institutions.

For facility monitoring, such as at hospitals, nursing homes, jails, and schools, grab samples are unlikely to provide representative information, because the wastewater samples are likely to be highly variable due to the shedding dynamics of the small number of individuals contributing to the samples and lack of mixing, which usually occurs in the many kilometers of pipes leading to a treatment plant. Thus, grab sampling at facilities will result in data with a higher likelihood of false negatives, and negative results need to be weighed against the probability of detecting a signal with a particular sampling method. For example, even composite samplers collect only a small subset of the wastewater discharged and could miss a single case within a facility. Passive sampling, described below, holds promise as a way to integrate and concentrate facility samples over time, for sites where presence/absence data are sufficient. Special considerations regarding facility data sharing to address the heightened risk of stigmatization and reidentification that attaches to smaller-scale sampling are discussed in Chapter 4.

Alternative Approaches in Development: Passive Sampling

Facility-level composite sampling may not be feasible or cost-effective to deploy and maintain. In facilities, passive sampling represents a significant improvement upon grab samples and may permit measurements at many more sites than composite sampling could accommodate (Bivins et al., 2022). Passive samplers are designed to capture the target organism from wastewater as the wastewater stream passes over or through the sampler, concentrating the target in situ over the time period of deployment. Passive samplers have been used to monitor for microorganisms, such *Salmonella Typhi* B (Sikorski and Levine, 2020), as well chemical contaminants that are at low levels in the environment (Godlewska, 2021), but most of the recent work with passive samplers has been to detect SARS-CoV-2 virus. Recent studies have focused on evaluating different material for capture of the virus, including cotton buds, cotton gauze (e.g., Moore swabs), cellulose sponges, electronegative membranes, and granular activated carbon (Bivins et al., 2022; Hayes et al., 2022) as well as novel housings to hold different materials (Hayes et al., 2021; Schang et al., 2020). Benefits of passive samplers include their low cost and ease of placement without the need for secure locations or electricity for composite samplers, which may facilitate measurements at many more sites than composite sampling could accommodate (Bivins et al., 2022). However, sampling personnel need to visit a site twice per sample for placement and retrieval.

Passive samplers generally produce qualitative data (i.e., presence/absence), but semi-quantitative data are feasible with accompanying adsorption isotherm data. Passive samplers have the potential to increase the sensitivity of detection because larger volumes of wastewater can be exposed to the sampler compared to the limited sample volume (generally <100 mL) used in laboratory concentration methods. Greater sensitivity of passive samplers over traditional sampling has been reported, particularly when SARS-CoV-2 concentrations in wastewater were <1 gene copy/mL (Schang, 2021). In facilities such as hospitals and nursing homes, which may have large variability in viral concentrations in wastewater across grab samples, passive sampling represents a significant improvement (Bivins et al., 2022). The amount of target organisms detected is affected by many factors, including the waste-stream characteristics (e.g., flow, solids), the efficiency of attachment, the time the sampler is deployed, the saturation point of the material used, flow through the sampler device, and analytical recovery from the material used in the sampler (Bivins et al., 2022). Researchers have reported linear accumulation of SARS-CoV-2 over specific time frames (10–48 hours) (Habtewold et al., 2022; Hayes et al., 2022), but the complexity of the adsorption dynamics makes it difficult to relate empirical concentrations from passive samplers to the data currently being generated from batch or composite liquid samples. Deployment across a large sewershed has been shown to reflect the spatiotemporal SARS-CoV-2 clusters across a city (Li et al., 2022).

Application of passive samplers is currently limited to qualitative or semi-quantitative needs and not appropriate for wastewater treatment plant sampling in NWSS. This type of sampler is useful when detecting the presence of a pathogen is important, such as determining spread during an epidemic or identification of a rare emerging pathogen (see Chapter 6). Additional research and development could advance passive sampling toward more quantitative applications. This will require a greater understanding of the efficacy of partitioning over time to different materials in different wastewater system conditions as well as the efficiency of recovering the nucleic acids from the sampler material. Research should also examine different types of target organisms, such as enveloped or nonenveloped viruses, Gram-negative or Gram-positive bacteria, and yeasts (e.g., *Candida auris*).

Sample Handling

Proper handling and storage of wastewater surveillance samples are crucial to produce accurate and reliable data. In wastewater without proper storage, coronaviruses experience rapid decay, with a 99.9 percent reduction in titer occurring within 2–4 days (Simpson et al., 2021). The Association of Public Health Laboratories (APHL, 2022) and CDC[2] have developed guidance for sample handling in wastewater surveillance based on enveloped viruses, such as SARS-CoV-2. Both APHL (2022) and CDC recommend that wastewater samples be stored at 4°C until processing, unless immediate processing is possible. APHL (2022) recommends storing for no longer than 4 days, while CDC suggests that if processing of samples is delayed more than 24 hours after collection, the sample should be spiked with a matrix recovery control (see Chapter 3) before refrigerating it at 4°C or freezing it at –20°C or –70°C. However, several studies caution against storing untreated bulk wastewater samples at lower temperatures, specifically –20° and –80°C, based on observed decreases in viral load (Ahmed et al., 2020; Huge et al., 2022). NWSS does not require specific sample handling procedures.

Different pathogens are likely to have different survival times under various storage conditions, and these storage effects on recovery need to be

---

[2] See https://www.cdc.gov/nwss/testing.html.

understood. Additionally, it is important to understand the variability introduced by different approaches in storage to determine whether increased consistency of methods should be required. Issues associated with sample archiving are discussed in Chapter 3.

Technical Developments for Sampling

Looking forward, wastewater surveillance is rapidly becoming part of the public health system, and as facilities are designed and built or renovated in the future, improved access to the wastewater system will simplify logistics and make representative sampling simpler. Logistics are often more challenging than technology gaps, and engineering adaptations to wastewater plumbing might overcome some of the barriers to collecting samples at facilities. Sampling ports on new facilities could be designed to access points in the system best suited for capturing a well-mixed sample that includes the entire facility.

New technologies can also improve how samples are collected or how data are interpreted. "Smart" manholes could also be used to capture ancillary measurements that aid in interpretation of sample data. For example, the City of Houston has approximately 2,300 smart manhole covers; most measure depth to wastewater in the manhole. A limited number of the smart manhole covers also measure flow velocity (Wolken et al., 2023). Flow is used to normalize the amount of waste passing a sample site, but in pipes that are only partially filled, this is very difficult to measure, adding to the uncertainty of how much of a daily average waste stream a sample might represent or how much was captured on a grab sample. Apart from smart manholes, other developing technologies can more accurately measure flows in smaller pipes that are only partially full. These data are valuable for interpreting sample concentrations and estimating how much of a facility's waste stream was captured.

CONCLUSIONS AND RECOMMENDATIONS

To be most actionable and reliable, a national wastewater surveillance system should use representative sampling methods and move toward consistent sampling at all participating long-term sampling sites. Representative sampling methods are considered those that effectively capture waste input from a community over a given time period. At most sites, this would mean flow-weighted composite samples of wastewater influent. Solids sampling is also a promising strategy, although more characterization is needed on the time frame of inflows that are represented by solids sampling (compared to liquid composite samples of the inflow) and methods to ensure consistency and comparability. Small or low-resourced communities may need additional support to provide composite samplers or staff to maintain the equipment, but such investments are worthwhile to ensure useful data from the surveillance effort. Over the next 5–8 years, CDC should work to move the program toward consistent sampling methods and procedures to reduce a source of variability and improve comparability, including training for sampling personnel.

For rapid trend resolution in support of public health action, nearly all wastewater surveillance systems should sample at least twice per week for RSV, influenza, and SARS-CoV-2, but additional data analysis will be necessary to determine appropriate sampling intervals for other targets added. Ultimately, the inherent variability in a given pathogen target and the intended use of those data will determine the temporal sampling needs. For respiratory viruses, twice-weekly sampling is sufficient to determine trends, although dense sampling networks (e.g., Houston's 39 wastewater treatment plants) may possibly provide enough confirmation of trends such that weekly sampling is sufficient. During an outbreak, increased frequency of sampling would allow localities to react to trends more quickly. Trade-offs may need to be assessed between setting different sampling frequencies as needed for different pathogens versus consistent sampling frequency for all targets (and which targets would dictate the overall sampling frequency). Less frequent sampling may be appropriate for use cases other than tracking trends of endemic pathogens (e.g., occasional measurements to assess levels in a community).

CDC should provide technical support for state and local optimization of sampling sites to maximize the value of NWSS data based on local, state, and national public health objectives and enhance the program's sustainability. Some initial statistical methods are available that can be used to evaluate the redundancy of existing sites and the value of new sampling locations to ensure that the range of demographics are appropriately included. To support these efforts, CDC should convene centralized expertise as a resource for states to formulate adaptive sampling and data analytics strategies. As the suite of core wastewater surveillance targets expands and pathogens evolve, these analyses will need to be revisited.

In a holistic wastewater surveillance system, facility sampling (e.g., nursing homes, hospitals, correctional facilities) should be part of a diversified approach that also benefits especially vulnerable populations. Facility-based testing would be a more effective mode of sampling compared to community-wide wastewater surveillance to understand spatial spread and trends in antibiotic resistance and specific pathogens such as *Candida auris*, which have significant health impacts at hospitals, skilled nursing facilities, and assisted living facilities. As opposed to sampling at more aggregated sites, such as centralized wastewater treatment plants, facility monitoring is likely to produce clear actionable information needed to contain localized outbreaks and inform facility-based prevention, particularly when data are correlated to clinical laboratory and health outcome data. For example, significant changes in the frequency of detection of antibiotic resistance genes above a certain threshold in facility wastewater can provide an early warning signal for potential spread or new infections and prompt facility-based epidemiological follow-up. For targets beyond antibiotic resistance, CDC, states, and localities will need to decide the benefits of other facility monitoring when balancing wastewater surveillance investments to support public health goals. Advances in passive sampling are promising and may make facility sampling increasingly cost-effective.

Research and development to improve sampling data quality and comparability is needed to increase the value of the data collected. Research needs include the following:

- **Optimization of sampling methods to ensure a representative sample and reduce variability.** There will always be an irreducible minimum variability in pathogens due to the stochastic nature of their occurrence and the chance of capture when sampling small volumes relative to the system as a whole. Research and development of methods targeted to reduce additional variability to the intrinsic minimum would enable better characterization of pathogen occurrence. This research can then be used to inform decisions to promote more consistency across NWSS or, at minimum, determine comparable methods.
- **Development and validation of passive samplers.** Specific studies should be conducted to determine sensitivity (i.e., ability to detect low levels of target) and compare passive sampler capture over time with traditional composite sampling to evaluate the ability to produce quantitative or semi-quantitative results in different waste streams to aid in the interpretation of results.
- **Comparison of solid versus liquid sampling.** Additional research is needed to compare the effectiveness of both sampling methods for reducing sampling-derived variability and improving comparability across sites. Research is also needed to define the representativeness of various solid sampling approaches in different wastewater treatment systems, and if and where system configurations may be inappropriate for representative solids sampling.
- **Statistical analysis of existing data to inform sampling optimization.** Additional research should be supported to develop standardized, validated approaches for optimizing sampling sites and identifying redundancies, thereby improving sustainability and cost-effectiveness.

- **Determination of a sampling strategy for new pathogen targets.** National analysis of NWSS sites and data on new targets are needed to gather information as to whether the new targets necessitate a different sampling frequency or spatial distribution to provide needed information while minimizing redundancy. This information is critical to inform decisions on trade-offs between sampling consistency across all targets and cost optimization alternatives.
- **Understanding and improving rural representation in NWSS.** Additional analyses of diverse data sets (e.g., cell phone data) could illuminate the extent to which existing NWSS sites encompass rural populations. Where critical data gaps exist, research could evaluate the feasibility of models to use existing site data to estimate disease trends in communities not included in the NWSS.

3

Analytical Methods and Quality Control for Endemic Pathogens

Appropriate analytical methods and quality control are central to producing reliable and interpretable data for national wastewater-based infectious disease surveillance. In this chapter, the committee discusses specific characteristics of analytical methods and associated quality criteria appropriate to a robust wastewater surveillance program for endemic pathogens and discusses technical constraints and opportunities. This chapter is focused on known endemic targets and polymerase chain reaction (PCR) methods that are likely to be used in the near term in the National Wastewater Surveillance System (NWSS) for endemic pathogen monitoring. Methods for emerging and unknown organisms are discussed in Chapter 6. The chapter begins with an overview of the state of analytical capacity for wastewater-based infectious disease surveillance, including sample processing, concentration, analysis, and storage, and then discusses opportunities for improving quality control. Research and development needs are also identified.

STATE OF ANALYTICAL CAPACITY

Current wastewater-based infectious disease surveillance efforts are hindered by significant data comparability issues. Myriad methods are employed to concentrate, detect, and quantify endemic pathogens, and the lack of consistency has led to a troubling amount of incomparable and sometimes unreliable data, complicating the interpretation and communication of findings (Ciannella et al., 2023). Data reliability was particularly a concern early in the pandemic as methods employed were evolving or inadequately validated, and some reliability issues remain today. Statistical analysis of the entire NWSS data set will prove difficult given these issues (Parkins et al., 2023).

As the NWSS program works to address these issues, additional targets are also being added, necessitating an understanding of the analytical specificity and sensitivity for the new targets. If the intent is to fit all targets into a single sample processing and analysis framework, which target and/or use case will determine the framework used? Different use cases and public health actions may require different workflows and pre-analytical sample processing strategies to generate actionable public health data. For instance, concentration, purification, and extraction methods optimized for viruses may result in suboptimal performance for bacterial or yeast targets. This may have implications in the sensitivity of the methods and whether they are "fit for purpose" for their intended use case. Differences in molecular detection methods may vary from target to target, particularly between RNA and DNA targets, but the variation in performance is unlikely in most cases to be significant relative to variability in concentration, purification, and extraction methods once optimized for a target (Wade et al., 2022).

Concentration, Extraction, and Purification Methods

Understanding performance in the stages of concentration, extraction, and purification are pivotal in the pre-analytical sample processing for wastewater surveillance. A variety of different methods have been evaluated for either liquid or solid samples, each with its strengths and limitations (see Figure 3-1) (Ciannella et al., 2023; Pecson et al 2021; Philo et al., 2021; Chik et al., 2021; Rusinol et al., 2020). No current approach has been identified as optimum for both solids and liquids. In addition to the impact on PCR-based detection, concentration and extraction can impact sequencing methods (Hielmso et al.,2017).

Methods may vary significantly in performance across targets and different matrices. For example, filtration and ultrafiltration methods are often used to concentrate viruses in liquids based on adsorption or size exclusion, respectively, whereas centrifugation may be instrumental for concentrating bacteria and protozoa via density differences. Chemical flocculation or precipitation techniques can also be used to concentrate particles, thereby increasing the yield of target pathogens for analytical purposes. The efficacy of these methods can be variable, influenced by factors such as the pathogen target, the wastewater matrix (e.g., liquid versus solid phase, pretreatment level, age) and the chemical composition of samples (see Figure 3-2) (Pecson et al., 2021; Zahedi et al., 2021). Further, the study methodologies for comparing concentration methods varies between studies, with different target organisms, methods and matrices. North and Bibby (2023)

Sample processing and extraction:

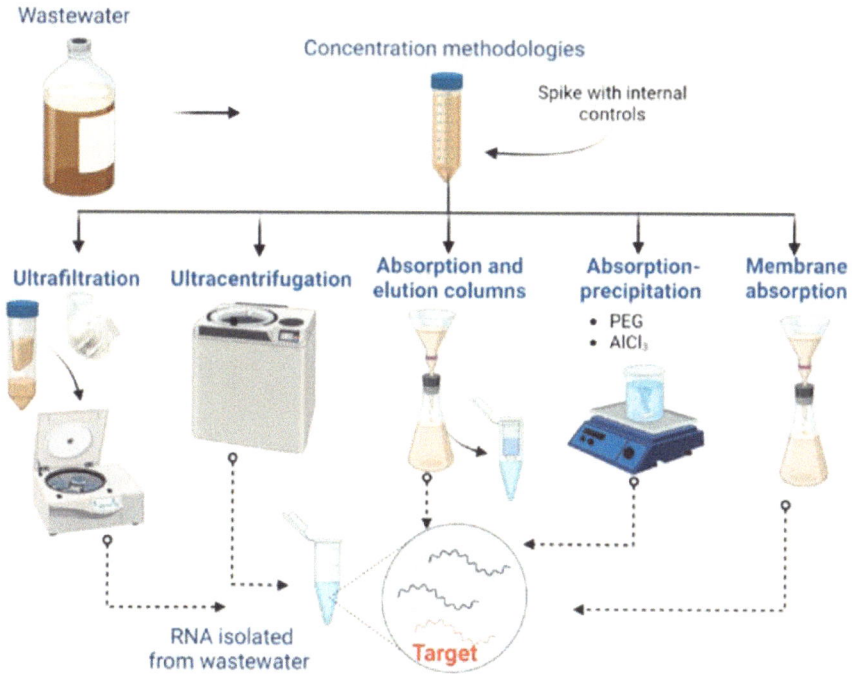

FIGURE 3-1 Many concentration methods are currently used for wastewater-based infectious disease surveillance.
SOURCE: Parkins et al., 2023.

found concentration efficiencies for native targets were not representative of seeded targets, and that significant differences in method performance was demonstrated across native targets. Identification of the most effective concentration methods would require additional studies using a consistent study design, set of targets, and wastewater matrices across an array of wastewater samples.

In the extraction step that follows concentration in wastewater surveillance for SARS-CoV-2, the selection of reagents and kits is pivotal to the isolation of nucleic acids from the concentrated sample. The efficiency and variability of these methods for a single target, but also between targets, can significantly impact the purity and quantity of the recovered genetic material, making comparability between methods difficult to interpret. In research exploring the variability among samples from the same site collected at different times during the same day for SARS-CoV-2 RNA in wastewater, Bivins et al. (2021) noted that process recovery efficiency

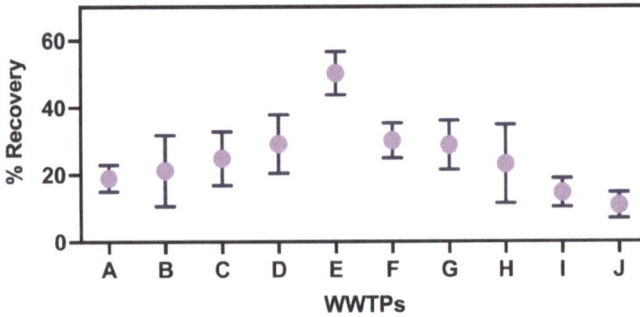

FIGURE 3-2 Recovery (mean ± standard deviation) of seeded SARS-CoV-2 RNA from 10 wastewater treatment plants (WWTPs A through J) using a single brand of concentrating pipette. Each WWTP was sampled three times.
SOURCE: Ahmed et al., 2022c.

was highly variable. Recent research efforts have shown that while commercially available extraction kits are widely used, the performance of various concentration and extraction procedures can vary significantly depending on the sample type and the presence of inhibitors (Bivins et al., 2021; Langan et al., 2022; Pérez-Cataluña et al., 2021; Steele et al., 2021). This necessitates careful selection and optimization of extraction methods for accurate wastewater-based epidemiology in COVID-19 surveillance. Furthermore, this variability calls for validation testing of commercial extraction kits using standardized samples and rapid dissemination of these results. Whitney et al. (2021) developed a kit-free extraction method, significantly enhancing RNA recovery efficiency, highlighting the potential of alternative approaches over traditional extraction kits.

Purification aims to alleviate the effects of inhibitors and other contaminants that could affect PCR amplification. Methods such as spin-column-based purification and bead-based magnetic separation are widely used (Ciannella et al., 2023). However, the efficiency of purification needs to be balanced against the potential loss of target nucleic acids, which is a trade-off that can affect sensitivity.

Without standardized concentration and extraction protocols, comparison of data between laboratories may be confounded (Servetas et al., 2022). Pecson et al. (2021) demonstrated the effect of different pre-treatment, concentration, extraction, and analysis methods across 32 different laboratories and 36 different standard operating procedures based on analysis of SARS-CoV-2 concentrations from replicates at a single wastewater treatment plant (see Figure 3-3). Eighty percent of the sample results were within a 2.3 log range (200-fold difference), but the authors also reported that recovery efficiency across the methods (determined by human coronavirus OC43

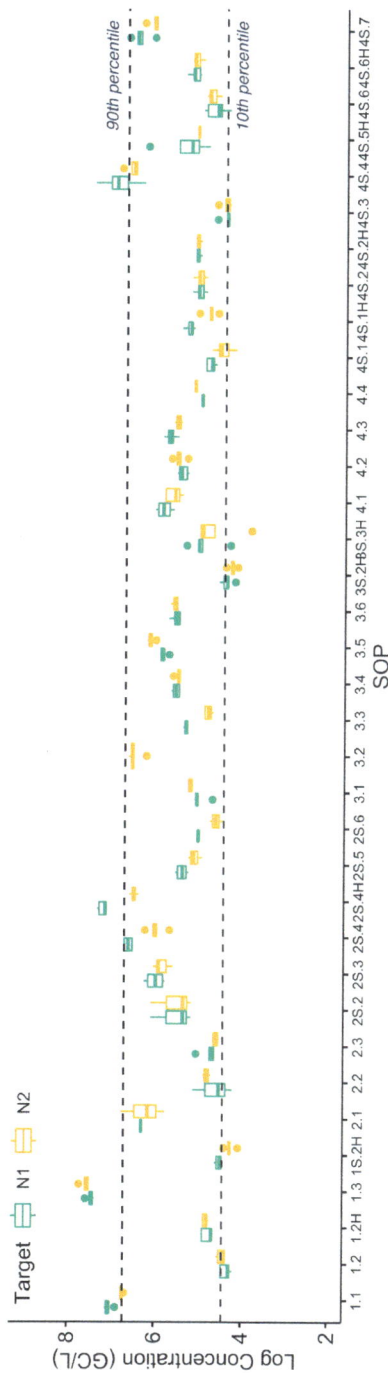

FIGURE 3-3 Recovery-corrected SARS-CoV-2 concentrations (N1 and N2 targets) for sample replicates from a single plant measured by 36 different standard operating procedures (SCPs). Nondetections and data excluded based on the quality control criteria are not plotted. The dashed lines show 10th and 90th percentiles across all results for both N1 and N2 primer/probe sets.
SOURCE: Pecson et al., 2021.

matrix spike) varied by seven orders of magnitude (10-million fold; Pecson et al., 2021). Additionally, variability between repeated runs of the same protocol can directly impact the quality and reliability of the PCR results, reducing confidence in the surveillance outputs and further complicating the task of comparative analyses across different jurisdictions.

Within the NWSS, there exists a significant diversity in the methods employed, reflective of the unique circumstances and capabilities of individual laboratories and the desire to be as inclusive as possible during the COVID-19 pandemic (Figure 3-4). As of May 2024, samples from 8.7 percent of NWSS sites were analyzed through a national testing contract, managed by Verily, which uses a single method for all sample processing and analysis, and 11.7 percent of NWSS sites were analyzed by WastewaterSCAN, which uses a different method (K. Cesa, CDC, personal communication, 2024). The remaining 80 percent of sites rely on individual public health laboratories that employ a diversity of methods. Feedback from local jurisdictions reveals an appreciation for the principle of standardization, but at the same time a reluctance to move away from their own established methods. This is due, in part, to concerns about being able to compare data from the new methods with the historical baseline, as well as an uncertainty about which methods are truly the best practices for their system, in light of the heterogeneous composition of wastewater across the nation. This preference underscores a tension between the need for standardized practices and the desire to maintain locally optimized methods. Development of a robust national wastewater surveillance system necessitates resolving this tension to ensure the production of reliable data that can be effectively compared across different programs, thereby facilitating more informed public health decisions. This resolution requires careful consideration of local needs and capabilities while striving for a level of standardization that enhances the overall quality and comparability of wastewater surveillance data.

As the demand for data from wastewater surveillance grows, there is an increasing need for the development of best practice guidelines that address the specific challenges of concentration, extraction, and purification in wastewater matrices (Ahmed et al., 2020; Servetas et al., 2022). Such guidelines should be informed by comparative studies that assess the performance of different methods under a variety of conditions, ultimately leading to a consensus on the most effective and reliable approaches for pathogen recovery prior to PCR analysis.

PCR Methods in Wastewater Surveillance

PCR techniques, specifically quantitative PCR (qPCR) and digital PCR (dPCR), are critical in wastewater surveillance for their ability to detect and quantify known pathogens with high sensitivity (see Figure 3-5). PCR-based methods use primers that are specific to the target strain, variant, or antibiotic resistance gene to select and amplify nucleic acid segments, enabling pathogen detection in wastewater at low concentrations. Standard PCR-based methods target DNA but can be combined with reverse transcription (RT) to target RNA; qPCR uses real-time monitoring of fluorescence over each amplification cycle (termed quantification cycle, C_q) to quantify the original target gene copies in the sample, relative to a standard curve (Kralik and Ricchi, 2017). Due to its speed and efficiency, qPCR is widely adopted allowing for the quantitative analysis of a large number of samples in a relatively short time frame. It is particularly effective for pathogens present at higher concentrations (Ahmed et al., 2022b; Ciesielski et al., 2021). However, qPCR's reliance on standard curves as a reference for quantification can be a limitation. Each time a new set of experiments is run, the standard curve must be meticulously recalibrated to ensure accuracy. This requirement for frequent recalibration introduces potential variability in the results, as slight differences in calibration can lead to different outcomes. The source of qPCR standards and how they are calibrated can vary significantly between laboratories and methods. The field lacks and would benefit from certified standards that are commercially available. This aspect of qPCR, while fundamental to its operation, can be a source of imprecision, especially when comparing results from different sets of experiments or different laboratories. Additionally, qPCR can be more susceptible than dPCR to inhibitors present in complex wastewater samples, which may affect its accuracy (Tiwari et al., 2022).

Unlike qPCR, dPCR provides absolute quantification by partitioning the sample into thousands of microreactions that are each measured by end-point fluorescence and enumerates based on a most probable number (MPN) statistical approach rather than requiring use of a standard curve. This feature reduces the impact of potential inhibitors and enhances the reliability and precision of the quantification, even in samples with low concentration targets in environmental samples with a high background of nontarget DNA (Ahmed et al., 2022b; Ciesielski et al., 2021). Droplet digital PCR (ddPCR), a subset of dPCR, further refines this process by using microdroplets to partition the sample, which allows for precise quantification in a highly reproducible manner. The high initial setup costs of dPCR can be a barrier to its widespread adoption. Typically dPCR also has a smaller dynamic range (about four orders of magnitude) and thus faces limitations when analyzing multiple targets simultaneously (i.e., multiplexing) with highly disparate concentrations in a sample. This can be overcome, however, if the expected range is known prior to the analysis, and adjusted via dilutions correction or through distribution in multiplex assays based on expected ranges. Additionally, recent advances in "next-generation"

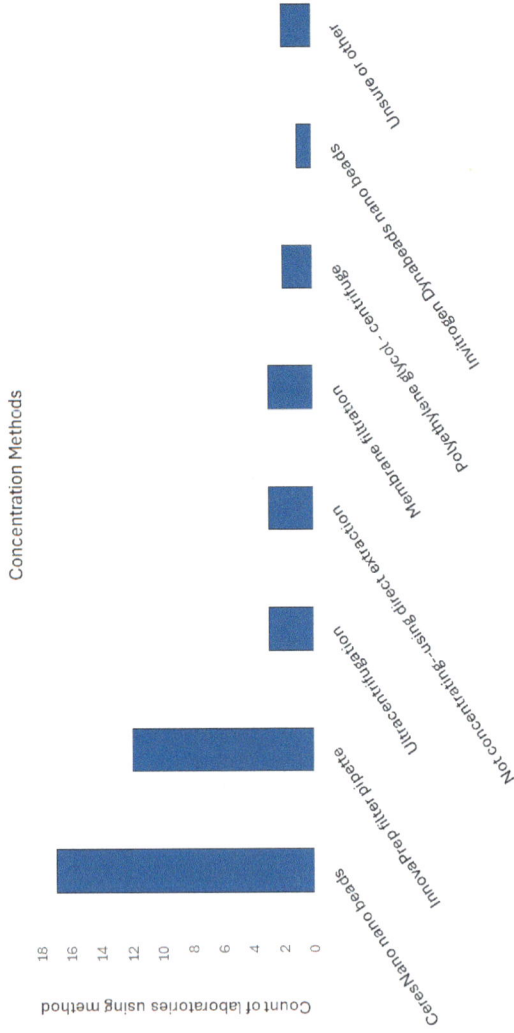

FIGURE 3-4 Results from an Association of Public Health Laboratories survey of concentration and extraction methods across analytical laboratories processing NWSS samples. Thirty-three laboratories responded.
SOURCE: Data from APHL, 2024.

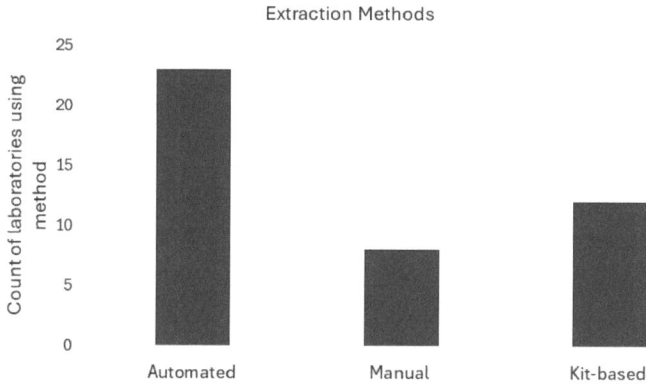

FIGURE 3-4 Continued

dPCR technology have reported increased dynamic range (six orders of magnitude; Jones et al., 2016; Shum et al., 2022).

Both qPCR and dPCR have been useful in wastewater-based infectious disease surveillance. Overall, the selection between these methods has generally depended on the specific requirements of the surveillance program, the available resources, and the intended use of the data. However, multiplexing in wastewater surveillance underscores the distinct attributes of qPCR and dPCR. When addressing the need for simultaneous detection of multiple targets within a sample, the efficiency of qPCR can be compromised. In multiplexing scenarios, the competition for reagents and primer-dimer formations can lead to reduced efficiency and accuracy in qPCR. In contrast, dPCR, with its quantification based on the MPN approach, is less impacted by these factors. Because dPCR partitions the sample into numerous micro-reactions, each individual reaction is less prone to the complexities and interferences seen in qPCR multiplexing. In addition, because each molecule of target is run in a separate droplet reaction, mismatches in the target with the primer or probe, such as with changing variants of SARS-CoV-2, can be visualized with some dPCR platforms (Schussman et al., 2022). This partitioning effectively isolates the reactions, ensuring that PCR efficiency does not significantly hinder the quantification process. This independence from reaction efficiency in dPCR, along with its enhanced resistance to inhibitors, makes it a more reliable and accurate choice for quantifying diverse targets in multiple assays. The recent advancements in dPCR technology, allowing for a broader dynamic range comparable to that of qPCR (Shum et al., 2022), further reinforce its applicability in multiplexing.

Despite the higher initial setup costs and the requirement for specialized expertise, the precision and reliability of dPCR in complex multiplex assays advocate for its increasing utility in wastewater surveillance. Recently, the NWSS recommended laboratories use dPCR, as opposed to qPCR, because dPCR is less subject to inhibition (Adams et al., 2024). Nevertheless, the strategic alignment of targets in multiplex assays, considering their concentration ranges and the nature of the targets (e.g., RNA vs. DNA, viral vs. bacterial) is an important consideration to ensure more consistent and reliable results across varied environmental samples. In minimizing the number of workflows, it may also be advantageous to couple pathogens with similar biochemical composition (e.g., coupling enveloped viruses together and coupling nonenveloped viruses together, or coupling DNA targets separately from RNA targets).

Biosafety and Laboratory Processing

One factor limiting the ability of laboratories to analyze wastewater pathogens is the necessity to adhere to biosafety protocols, which are determined based on the agent itself and the particular procedures to be undertaken. In the case of laboratories sampling wastewater for SARS-CoV-2 genetic material, which requires sample concentration as part of the testing, the Centers for Disease Control and Prevention (CDC) have indicated that enhanced biosafety level 2 (BSL-2) procedures are needed. This includes a BSL-2 laboratory with unidirectional airflow and use of respiratory protection and a separate designated area for putting on and taking off personal protective equipment.[1] CDC and the Water Environment Federation each have separate safety guidance for wastewater treatment plant workers sampling raw wastewater, including use of personal protective equipment (WEF, 2021).[2]

It should be recognized that, while BSL-2 laboratories are common, laboratories with certification at higher biosafety levels are less common and more expensive to design, operate, and conduct work in. Meanwhile, the concentration of pathogens in environmental samples (as opposed to clinical samples) is generally expected to be low, since in wastewater any human contributions are diluted with a large volume of carriage water in which the material is conveyed.[3] However, after concentration of samples, the genome concentration per unit volume in environmental samples could be in the same range as clinical samples, although with a much lower likelihood of containing viable organisms. As of the writing of this report, there has not been isolation of viable SARS-CoV-2 virus (as opposed to its genetic material) in municipal wastewater, and the presence and levels

---

[1] See https://www.cdc.gov/coronavirus/2019-ncov/lab/lab-biosafety-guidelines.html#environmental-testing.

[2] See https://www.cdc.gov/global-water-sanitation-hygiene/about/workers_handlingwaste.html#cdc_generic_section_2-personal-protective-equipment-ppe.

[3] An exception occurs when environmental samples are cultured for viable pathogens. In such cases, the levels of pathogens become higher.

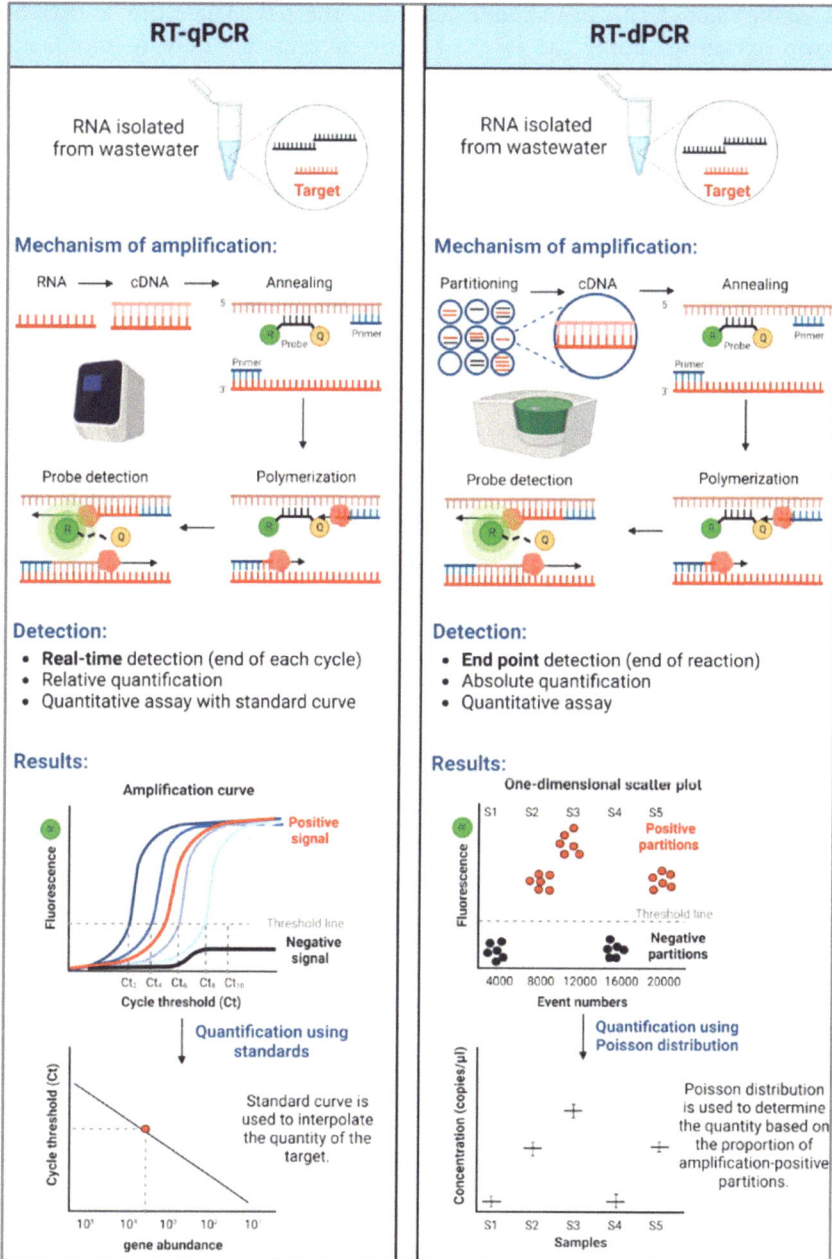

FIGURE 3-5 Processes of detection and quantification of gene targets using reverse transcription quantitative and digital PCR (RT-qPCR and RT-dPCR).
SOURCE: Parkins et al., 2023.

of viable microorganisms should determine the risk. Therefore, it may be inappropriate to apply the level of stringency in biosafety requirements for wastewater analyses that would be used for clinical laboratory work with the same pathogens if the risk does not justify the additional burdens posed by enhanced BSL-2. The World Health Organization (WHO) recently approved BSL-2 control measures for "non-propagative diagnostic laboratory work" on SARS-CoV-2, such as sequencing (WHO, 2024).

It may be feasible to confine higher hazard operations (and hence the need for a higher-biosafety-level laboratory) to a small footprint, for example by pasteurizing or otherwise inactivating samples. This may be feasible if molecular signatures of pathogens are the only end point to be examined. Some researchers have shown that pasteurization has reduced RNA recovery for SARS-CoV-2 (Islam et al., 2022; Robinson et al., 2022), while others have shown enhanced recovery (Cutrupi et al., 2023; Trujillo et al., 2021). The wastewater matrix has also been shown to influence the effect of pasteurization on RNA recovery (Beattie et al., 2022). More research is needed to determine optimal pasteurization methods for wastewater surveillance if enhanced BSL-2 conditions are expected to remain. Additionally, metadata on sample pretreatment are important because of these effects.

When other pathogens are added to the wastewater surveillance panel, either for endemic or emerging pathogens, a formal risk assessment should be conducted to assess the needed degree of biosafety required based on the proposed sampling and analysis protocols. Ideally, these analyses should be conducted well in advance so that wastewater surveillance can be implemented both safely and quickly for emerging pandemic threats. In addition, the effect of any pasteurization or inactivation process on ultimate method performance (specificity and sensitivity) needs to be evaluated for each target pathogen.

As additional biological knowledge and information about target pathogens is acquired, biosafety practices can and should be reassessed to ensure that they reflect the most current understanding of the biosafety risk. Given the evolving understanding of SARS-CoV-2 risks associated with wastewater surveillance, the biosafety handling regulations around SARS-CoV-2 should be reassessed to determine if enhanced BSL-2 procedures remain the appropriate handling guidance.

Sample Archiving

Short-term sample archiving is a necessary component of quality control in wastewater surveillance. Ideally, these samples would be archived for about 3 months to allow for reanalysis in case data anomalies or quality issues are raised. Retrospective investigation of infectious disease outbreaks could be facilitated by the existence of archived samples, as shown by

Teunis et al. (2004) with foodborne outbreaks. In most locations, short-term storage of concentrated, processed extracts for follow-up analysis would not require resources beyond those commonly found in analytical laboratories processing samples.

For a national wastewater surveillance program, a rotating, longer-term (multiyear) sample archive would be useful for understanding clusters of illness that may become apparent. Long-term archiving would not be necessary at every site or even every state. At a national scale, wastewater surveillance sites from several large cities across the country could be identified as key sites for long-term storage. Development of several longer-term archives would likely require purchase of additional -80°C freezers at those select locations.

CDC recommends that processed, concentrated wastewater surveillance samples be archived at -70°C,[4] and the Association of Public Health Laboratories recommends storage at -80°C (AHPL, 2022). Raw, unprocessed samples are not typically recommended for archiving because of the large storage space required by raw samples as well as the effect of the freeze-thaw cycle on RNA recovery (Markt et al., 2021). Research suggests that longer-term (35–122 days) freezing of raw wastewater solids also reduced RNA measurements by an average of 60 percent (Simpson et al., 2021). Stability of RNA concentrated on filters after sample processing proved more promising and showed improved recovery after 19 days of storage at -80°C (Beattie et al., 2022). Yet, the integrity of RNA for long-term storage remains poorly understood. Different pathogens are likely to have different survival times under various storage conditions, and these storage effects on recovery need to be understood.

An in-depth research initiative is needed to refine and optimize the process for long-term archiving of wastewater samples. Research should examine best practices for long-term sample integrity at all stages of sample processing, including removal of solid particles and concentration of the microbial fraction (e.g., centrifugation, filtration), use of RNA stabilization solutions or reagents and their implication on downstream analytical methods, and rapid freezing protocols that prevent RNA degradation. Quality control considerations should also be included, such as sample homogenization methods (including even distribution of any stabilizing agent) and best practices for aliquoting the stabilized samples into small volumes. There is a need to develop a protocol for initial quality control checks, such as utilizing qPCR or dPCR to assess RNA integrity prior to storage, which will then serve as a critical baseline for subsequent periodic evaluations to ensure continued sample integrity over time. The research should also determine an ideal long-term storage duration that optimizes space efficiency without

---

[4] See https://www.cdc.gov/nwss/sampling.html.

compromising the integrity of the samples. Establishing a regular monitoring schedule to evaluate the integrity of the stored nucleic acids is vital for enabling timely interventions in the event of degradation. Collectively, these research needs should provide a thorough understanding of each step in the long-term archiving process.

Long-term archiving of wastewater samples also raises questions about what sorts of future analyses utilizing these samples are ethically acceptable. Analyses may, for instance, explore targets that were unknown at the time of sample collection and that contributing communities may view as involving potential stigmatization. In Chapter 4, the committee describes how an ethics advisory body could be helpful in weighing the risks and benefits of proposed secondary uses of NWSS digital data. This body could perform the same work for stored samples.

OPPORTUNITIES TO IMPROVE DATA UTILITY

There are opportunities for improving both data quality and data comparability to enhance the utility of NWSS data. Opportunities to improve data quality involve improving accuracy and precision of data within any given laboratory (intralaboratory). Opportunities for improving data comparability involve steps to characterize and minimize interlaboratory differences in methods or technical implementation of the methods so that data are comparable and relatable for a broader interpretation of the data regionally and nationally.

Improving Intralaboratory Data Quality

Quality data are essential for reliable interpretation and public health decision making. Within each laboratory, good data quality is important to the reliability of individual sample measurements and facilitates the interpretation of trends for repeated samples from a given site. Good intralaboratory data quality also strengthens the ability to compare the analytical results among different sites analyzed by a single laboratory.

Improving intralaboratory data quality decreases the inaccuracy and imprecision that may arise at any stage of the process, from sample storage to concentration method, RNA/DNA extraction, and PCR amplification. Data inaccuracies and imprecision can be associated with a wide range of sources including small deviations in the method protocol, instrument error, reagent variability, and analyst practices. As an example, it is well known that diverse extraction methods contribute to data variability (Figure 3-3). The data variability observed in one step can be amplified by subsequent steps in processing. For example, the extraction step directly affects the yield and purity of nucleic acids and, consequently, the resulting impurities can impact the PCR reactions (Ahmed et al., 2022c). The following sections discuss several opportunities to improve the precision of measurements within a laboratory and also minimize intralaboratory variability: SOPs, robust quality assurance and quality control (QA/QC), analyst training and proficiency testing, and proper calibration and maintenance of laboratory equipment.

Development of, Validation of, and Adherence to SOPs

A best practice is that each laboratory developing or adopting a wastewater surveillance pipeline should take pains to vigorously evaluate the performance of its methods and validate its application to the types of samples that it receives. Detailed written SOPs specific to the laboratory should be developed for each method in a control chain with explicit details on procedures, reagents, instruments, safety, contraindications, etc., and this information should be made available to provide context for the measurements and aid in understanding observed differences. Deviations from SOPs should be discouraged for all samples, but recorded if they occur. Strict adherence to SOPs will help minimize variability between replicate samples. When a laboratory adopts a new method, initial precision recovery studies should be performed on seeded samples to understand the accuracy and precision. Further, ongoing precision recovery studies should be performed regularly to ensure method performance does not change over time. Matrix spike samples should be processed whenever new sites are brought online or when changes in the wastewater matrix occur to ensure that matrix effects do not adversely impact performance of the methods.

Each new pathogen target added to the wastewater surveillance panel (see Chapter 5) will require development of validated assays that demonstrate high sensitivity and specificity in wastewater to produce data that are both robust and reliable. Many pathogen assays have been developed for the clinical setting, and these assays will need to be demonstrated to work with environmental samples. For targets intended to be implemented nationally, CDC should harness the expertise of the NWSS Centers of Excellence and foster collaborations with academia and commercial interests to develop validated assays that meet performance criteria. Best practices for primer design for PCR assays include robust *in silico* analysis and performance testing designed to reduce the likelihood of false positives and increase the efficiency of PCR amplification. For targets that may have a more regional implementation, NWSS should define sensitivity and specificity guidelines to ensure that assays target relevant organisms, strains, or variants with the most current genomic sequences. In addition to assay validation, CDC, with assistance from the National Institute of Standards and Technology (NIST) or other appropriate national and international standard-setting bodies, should recommend appropriate standards and spike control materials that can simulate the behavior of the target pathogens in wastewater and provide a reliable benchmark for assay performance.

Robust QA/QC

Minimum criteria for data inclusion that are aligned with the latest standards in PCR data generation and reporting are necessary to ensure quality data in a robust national wastewater surveillance system. These criteria include mandated use of standardized controls, reference materials, and calibration procedures that can be applied universally across various PCR platforms. Existing comprehensive guidelines and standards, such as the Minimum Information for Publication of Quantitative Real-Time PCR Experiments (MIQE) guidelines (Bustin et al., 2009), its digital counterpart for dPCR (Huggett et al., 2013), and the Environmental Microbiology Minimum Information (EMMI) guidelines (Borchardt et al., 2021), provide a robust foundation for such a standardization effort. These documents should serve not merely as recommendations but as keystones in laboratory practice. Based on these established guidelines, NWSS should require the following as minimum criteria for data inclusion: use of proper performance controls, control verification, and performance limits for diagnostic assays. Results of these QA/QC steps should be reported as metadata along with data submission.

Use of proper performance controls. Incorporation of appropriate seeded controls to assess total method recovery as a standard best practice helps in monitoring the efficiency of the sample processing pipeline and ensures performance as intended. Additional seeded controls may be warranted to evaluate performance of individual procedures within the sample processing pipeline (e.g., nucleic acid extraction recovery controls). In addition to the pathogen targets, performance controls for normalization targets should also be included (e.g., pepper mild mottle virus, CrAssphage [*Carjivirus communis*]; see Chapter 4) because the quantities of these targets are often incorporated in wastewater surveillance data. Seeded controls should be validated in parallel to intended targets during initial precision recovery studies to ensure adequacy as an indicator of performance.

Control verification. Inclusion of appropriate positive and negative controls is essential to demonstrate the integrity of analysis. Data should only be included in NWSS if positive and negative controls behave as expected in every assay run, with positive controls confirming assay functionality and negative controls ensuring the absence of contamination. Use of inhibition controls should be required to minimize false negatives and evaluate effect on quantitation. Inhibition controls should consist of the target nucleic acids, because different assays can exhibit different levels of inhibition. Inhibition control tests should be conducted at new locations and when wastewater characteristics change at a specific plant.

Performance limits for diagnostic assays. Laboratories should validate and report the lower limit of detection (LOD) and the limit of quantitation (LOQ) for each assay used in their program, because these limits are essential for interpreting the significance of low-level detections. The MIQE guidelines (Bustin et al., 2009) and the EMMI guidelines (Borchardt et al., 2021) provide robust frameworks for defining these thresholds. According to these guidelines, LOD is commonly described as the lowest concentration detected with statistical significance using a given procedure or instrument, while LOQ refers to the lowest concentration at which the analyte can be quantitatively determined with acceptable precision and accuracy. According to these guidelines, analysts should perform rigorous validation studies, including the use of standard curves and control materials, to establish these limits for each assay. Standardizing the definition and determination of LOD and LOQ across laboratories will help minimize variability and ensure the reliability of surveillance data. Multiplexing should focus on targets that are expected to be in a similar range.

Analyst Training and Proficiency Testing

Education and training for laboratory personnel, emphasizing the importance of maintaining high-quality standards and following established protocols, are central to data quality. This should include the establishment of benchmarking and regular proficiency testing, enabling laboratories to gauge and calibrate their methods against standardized metrics. Records of personnel training and proficiency testing should be maintained and updated.

Proper Calibration and Maintenance of Instruments and Laboratory Equipment

Inadequate or lack of calibration for laboratory instruments and equipment can be a significant source of uncontrolled variability. This is especially the case if multiple similar instruments (e.g., PCR thermocylers, pipettors) are used interchangeably. Rigorous maintenance and calibration programs should be employed to ensure proper function and quantification, and any deviation from the regular schedule should be recorded.

Improving Interlaboratory Comparability

Maximizing data comparability between laboratories involves not only the data quality issues discussed in the previous section but other greater sources of variability, such as disparate methodologies implemented by different laboratories and differences inherent in the samples each laboratory receives (e.g., from vastly different systems, different types of samples; see Chapter 2). As additional targets are added to wastewater surveillance (see Chapter 5), the selection of sample processing methods is likely to reflect a prioritization of some targets over others, and these priorities may differ among public health jurisdictions. As with intralaboratory data quality, there are opportunities to minimize interlaboratory variability, although some variability is inherent that cannot easily be reduced. There are four main options to minimize interlaboratory variability: (1) defining explicit sample and performance acceptance criteria, (2) limiting methods only to those that perform as well as an approved reference method, (3) developing a standard method, and (4) normalization.

Defining Acceptance Criteria for Samples and Analytical Performance

Definition of explicit performance criteria for a method (e.g., defining the range of acceptable recovery, the lower limit of detection, or limit of quantification) can help to minimize interlaboratory variability. Definition of these types of parameters can allow laboratories the choice to select methods that will work in their setting while maintaining expectations on performance. This is perhaps the least restrictive approach to minimizing interlaboratory differences. Incentivization programs could be implemented to encourage laboratories to consistently meet or surpass these standards.

To improve comparability, the NWSS, in partnership with other standard-setting bodies or organizations, could also establish specific definitions for the equivalent sample volumes or effective sample volumes, which can control for different inputs into a diagnostic assay, accounting for differences in pre-analytical processing. The effective sample volume relates to the proportion of the original sample that is interrogated by the diagnostic assay (Fung et al., 2020). Equivalent sample volumes refer to the original sample volume that is analyzed in each PCR, accounting for sample processing (Crank et al., 2023). Research is needed to define the equivalent and effective sample volume necessary to meet NWSS quality objectives for their intended use cases for each target. Establishing effective and equivalent sample volumes is crucial as they directly influence the limit of detection and the overall interpretability of surveillance findings.

Requiring Performance Equivalent to Validated Reference Methods

A second approach would to be to establish a "gold standard" reference method by which to compare other methods. The reference method would be selected by CDC or the Centers of Excellence to meet performance criteria supportive of the designated use of the data for a particular target. Other methods could then be evaluated for equivalency to the reference against a performance panel. Once demonstrated equivalent, the other methods could be used by laboratories if it better meets their needs. The benefit of this approach is that the universe of methods is narrowed and flexibility is provided to the laboratories to select methods that work with their instrument platforms, experience, and other local conditions. Alternatively, CDC could maintain a limited list of approved and acceptable methods that have been designated as equivalent and/or fit for purpose. This is similar to how WHO has handled methods for polio surveillance.

Requiring Standard Methods

Standardization of all components of sample processing and analysis would seem to offer the greatest ability to minimize variability between laboratories. However, this is also the most onerous approach to accomplish and still would not fully control sources of variability between laboratories. Variability due to matrix effect, system differences, and analyst precision would not be adequately controlled by this standardization approach, and there is concern that differences among wastewater treatment plants may necessitate different methods. Further, forcing laboratories toward a single approach could limit adoption of the method for a variety of issues, such as experience with alternative methods, cost, and available instrumentation. Full standardization may also stifle scientific advancement and engagement by the commercial and academic sectors.

If standardization is determined to be the best way to improve interlaboratory comparability, CDC could couple standardization efforts with the establishment of a centralized certification program for wastewater surveillance. Centralized training could support laboratories in transitioning to these standardized methods, fostering a more unified approach to wastewater surveillance across the board.

Data Normalization

A final option is to control for variability between laboratories during the data analysis and reporting phase through a carefully vetted data normalization process, which, as discussed in detail in Chapter 4, has yet to be identified. This approach is incumbent on well-validated methods and high-quality data for all laboratories involved, but, ideally, data normalization could adjust for differences in analytical methods used or system characteristics. Further discussion of normalization can be found in Chapter 4.

A Way Forward

A thorough analysis of existing data and methods used can help determine whether a limited number of sample processing and analytical approaches can achieve adequate data quality to achieve data comparability objectives for the NWSS. However, such analyses require metadata on pre-analytical and analytical methods and controls (and similar reporting as required by EMMI guidelines) be provided along with reported results. The reporting requirements need to be detailed enough to identify slight differences in the applications of the same method across different laboratories. The integration of artificial intelligence and machine learning should help analyze large data sets to identify the largest sources of variability (see Chapter 4). NWSS may also benefit from lessons learned from ongoing research at the Environmental Protection Agency Office of Research and Development, which is working to develop comparable PCR methods (a standard method and/or performance metrics) for viable pathogens in wastewater to better understand recreational exposure risks and potential drinking water effects.

Once the sources of data variability are well understood, CDC will need to determine the best strategy from those listed above to ensure the production of reliable data that can be effectively compared across the NWSS platform, thereby facilitating more informed public health decisions. This decision requires careful consideration of local needs and capabilities while striving for a level of standardization that enhances the overall quality and comparability of wastewater surveillance data.

Looking Ahead

Technology development offers potential for further improving data quality in wastewater surveillance analysis. For example, support for technologies that automate and standardize steps within the PCR process, including liquid handling, concentration, extraction, and purification, could potentially reduce human sources of error and variability. Innovation in real-time sampling and analysis technologies could spark a quantum leap in wastewater surveillance. The immediacy with which data can be acquired paves the way for a more nimble and precise response to emergent public health threats, an attribute that is indispensable for the early detection and containment of infectious diseases. The sophistication of real-time analysis tools lies in their ability to detect a broader spectrum of pathogens and substances, including those at lower concentrations that might elude traditional methods. As these technologies evolve to become more user friendly, their application could expand into varied environments, bridging the gap in public health surveillance capabilities, particularly in resource-constrained settings. Such democratization of health monitoring tools is vital for equitable public health interventions.

CONCLUSIONS AND RECOMMENDATIONS

The observed diversity and the lack of standardization in analytical methodologies for wastewater surveillance have led to significant variability and decreased comparability of data from different sites. The wastewater surveillance system developed through rapid research and innovation, and the resulting interlaboratory variability in methods for extraction, purification, amplification, and data reporting, limits understanding of trends in pathogen concentrations across sites. A wastewater surveillance system with comparable data will better support effective public health interventions at regional and national scales.

Rigorous data analysis efforts are needed to determine whether a single standardized analytical method is necessary to improve NWSS comparability or whether other approaches are reasonable. To minimize interlaboratory variability, the committee identified four alternative strategies: (1) defining acceptance criteria for performance, (2) limiting methods only to those that perform as well as an approved reference method, (3) developing a standard method, and (4) using as yet undiscovered data normalization approaches. Research on the sources of variability in sample processing and analysis is essential to identify the best alternative (or some combination) to improve comparability while balancing associated trade-offs. Full method standardization for sample processing and analysis could offer the greatest ability to minimize interlaboratory variability but it may also stifle scientific advancement.

Rigorous quality control standards should be developed to increase the reliability and interpretability of NWSS data. The NWSS should enforce criteria for data inclusion, including standardized controls, reference materials, and calibration procedures. The committee recommends several best practices for reducing intralaboratory variability, including development and adherence to SOPs that are made available to others, adoption of widely recognized QA/QC guidelines to ensure data consistency and integrity, use of performance controls, and use of positive and negative controls. Additionally, establishing a centralized certification program for wastewater surveillance laboratories, including benchmarking and proficiency testing programs, will align wastewater surveillance methods with these standards. CDC and its Centers of Excellence should develop validated assays for current and new targets with defined sensitivity and specificity. By spearheading these validation efforts and setting forth recommendations for standard materials, spike controls, and equivalent and effective sample volume parameters, CDC, with assistance from NIST and other standard-setting bodies, can bolster the consistency and comparability of data across surveillance efforts and also expedite the acceptance and integration of novel assays as new targets are added.

NWSS should develop a national system and guidelines for sample storage and invest in research to optimize long-term archiving for wastewater. In a national infectious disease wastewater surveillance system, short-term archiving (approximately 3 months) of all processed samples is essential for quality control, but several large sites should be identified for longer-term multiyear archiving. Several long-term archives would be valuable for retrospective analyses if a new pathogen is detected that was not previously analyzed. A regular monitoring schedule should be developed to assess the integrity of stored nucleic acids, enabling timely interventions if degradation is detected.

CDC should update its risk assessment for laboratories engaged in wastewater surveillance and re-evaluate the necessity of the biosafety level (BSL) 2 enhanced with BSL-3 precautions requirement. BSL-2 laboratories are common, but higher levels are less common and more expensive to design and operate. The understanding of the risks of SARS-CoV-2 in wastewater analyses has evolved with time, and future NWSS targets have been identified to inform an updated analysis, recognizing that the required biosafety level is a function of the pathogen, its concentration (and viable state), and the nature of the procedure being undertaken. BSLs applicable to clinical laboratories may not be appropriate for environmental laboratories because of differences in concentrations and laboratory procedures. WHO recently approved BSL-2 controls for nonpropagative laboratory analysis for SARS-CoV-2.

4

Data Analysis, Integration, and Interpretation for Endemic Pathogens

The National Wastewater Surveillance System (NWSS) currently collects weekly or semiweekly sampling data from over 1300 sites on SARS-CoV-2 viral levels, and some sites have recently expanded to collect other pathogens such as respiratory syncytial virus (RSV), influenza, norovirus, and Mpox. This system generates massive data with multiple sources of variability that challenge interpretation both within a single site and when trying to compare sites across a region or the nation. In addition to the inherent variability associated with wastewater system flows, different sampling and analysis processes and differences in the wastewater systems themselves (as discussed in Chapters 2 and 3) complicate comparison across sites. Amidst the many sources of variability, local, state, tribal, and national public health agencies work to discern trends and identify outbreaks to enhance knowledge and understanding and support public health action (see Figure 4-1). In this chapter, the committee reviews current strategies for data normalization, statistical and modeling methods, visualization tools, data integration, analytics, and disease forecasting and discusses challenges and opportunities for the next 5–8-year time frame. Recommendations for data sharing, which is central to support improvements in data reliability, comparability, and forecasting, are also presented.

DATA NORMALIZATION METHODS

Results from wastewater surveillance should accurately and precisely reflect what is happening with disease in the community so that the resulting data are interpretable and actionable. For example, if data accurately and

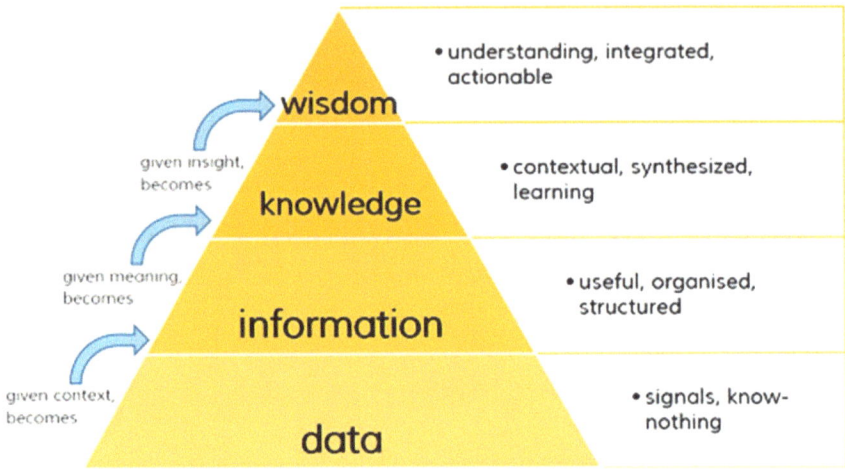

FIGURE 4-1 Converting data into knowledge and wisdom necessitates substantial efforts, such as data analysis and visualization tools for pattern recognition and learning, data integration across disparate data sets, and model-based disease forecasting to synthesize with other information to support public health action. SOURCE: Soloviev, 2016. https://creativecommons.org/licenses/by-nc-nd/4.0/.

precisely reflect disease burden in the community, then an uptick in measured wastewater concentrations can be interpreted as a rise in prevalence in the community. Furthermore, data that accurately and precisely reflect community disease burden facilitate the comparison of wastewater data between communities. For example, if neighboring counties exhibit different levels in their wastewater, local and state public health officials could interpret this as different levels of prevalence between the two communities.

As with any molecular measurements made from samples collected from the environment, inaccuracy, imprecision, and variability observed in the data stem from multiple sources, ranging from phenomena at the molecular level as the measurements are being analyzed to phenomena at the full wastewater system level, as discussed in Chapters 2 and 3. For example, at the molecular level, inaccuracies and variabilities might come from the efficiency and reproducibility of the nucleic acid extraction methods at recovering all of the target of interest. At the full system scale, variabilities could originate from wastewater being temporarily diluted during storm events.[1] Both of these examples can result in the observed absolute

---

[1] Combined sewer systems are designed to collect both rainwater and sanitary sewerage, which causes dilution from precipitation events. In separate sewer systems, which are more common, drainage from precipitation is designed to be collected via a distinct piping network, but there can still be significant infiltration and inflow, particularly in older systems, thereby allowing dilution of the wastewater (Lanning and Peterson, 2012).

abundances and trends not accurately reflecting the pathogen's prevalence in the community. Understanding and, when possible, correcting for these inaccuracies, imprecisions, and variabilities can improve data quality and interpretation.

Early in the COVID-19 pandemic, wastewater surveillance teams recognized the challenges that arise in measuring molecular targets in wastewater and ensuring the comparability of data produced from samples collected at different times and locations (Kumblathan et al., 2021). Indeed, comparing SARS-CoV-2 wastewater data across studies was complicated by the different sampling and measurement techniques as well as variable sewershed characteristics (Maere et al., 2022). Groups therefore sought approaches to address the imprecision, inaccuracies, and variabilities inherent in the measurements.

Normalization is a process of adjusting the measured wastewater concentrations to account for some of the underlying variables that impact inter- and intra-sewershed comparisons. Multiple normalization approaches have been applied to address different attributes. One common approach is using a factor that incorporates daily wastewater inflow rates. Theoretically, this approach addresses some of the variations observed within a single sewershed over time due to changes in wastewater input such as stormwater infiltration or irregular industrial inflows. Among the potential issues with this approach is that it requires wastewater treatment plants to share their daily flow data so that the analyzing laboratories can normalize their measurements. Although flow rates are routinely measured at larger wastewater treatment plants, the transfer of data can take time and, in some instances, even delay the posting or submitting of the wastewater surveillance data to larger reporting systems such as NWSS. Physio-chemical markers, such as electrical conductivity, have also been proposed to account for dilution effects (Langeveld et al., 2023; Wilde et al., 2022). Sewershed population is another normalizing factor that aims to address differences between sewersheds. Population values are typically reported as a constant (i.e., the residents of the sewershed) and do not address changing populations or people traveling into and out of the sewershed during the week and on weekends.

Other common normalizing approaches focus on the quantity of human excrement in the wastewater sample. These have included biological targets, such as human fecal indicator organisms, as well as chemical targets, such as ammonium, caffeine, paraxanthine, creatinine, and 5-hydroxyindoleacetic acid (Rainey et al., 2023). Of these, the fecal indicator viruses, including pepper mild mottle virus (PMMoV) and crAssphage [*Carjivirus communis*]-like viruses, are the most widely applied. Because these targets are ubiquitous in human fecal matter, they theoretically address temporal variability in a sewershed's wastewater fecal strength as well as inter-sewershed variability. Assuming that the recovery of the viral biomarkers through the sample preprocessing (e.g., polyethylene glycol precipitation) and nucleic acid extractions are reflective of the viruses targeted for wastewater-based epidemiology, using the biomarker targets also addresses variability in the recovery of viral nucleic acids from the wastewater samples.

There is presently no consensus with respect to which normalization factor performs best (Rainey et al., 2023). For relatively constant populations, the NWSS program currently recommends that viral concentration data from liquid samples be normalized by daily wastewater flow to account for changes in wastewater concentrations and to reduce variability in viral wastewater concentrations over time. For comparison across locations, NWSS recommends flow and population normalization to yield data in units of viral gene copies per person contributing to the sewershed per day. Finally, for solid samples, sites where flow rate data are not available, and populations that change substantially over time due to commuting, tourism, or other movement, the Centers for Disease Control and Prevention (CDC) suggests that it may be important to normalize with biological targets for human fecal normalization (CDC, 2023f). CDC advises that wastewater concentration data that have not been normalized may not yield meaningful differences in levels or direction and therefore cannot be compared across NWSS sites (CDC, 2023e).

A number of studies have assessed the value of normalization factors, with mixed results. To do this, researchers often look at correlations between clinical cases and wastewater concentrations that have or have not been normalized. For example, Wolfe et al. (2021) demonstrated that normalizing SARS-CoV-2 in primary sludge by concentrations of PMMoV RNA in solids was an effective approach when attempting to compare incidence of new laboratory-confirmed COVID-19 cases across wastewater treatment plant sites. Ai et al. (2021), however, found that normalizing influent SARS-CoV-2 measurements by PMMoV or crAssphage (*Carjivirus communis*) did not improve correlations. The mixed results on normalization are likely largely attributable to distinctive aspects of the methods applied and the specific samples. Indeed, a notable challenge in using molecular or chemical measurements to normalize some cases is that normalizing may actually increase the overall error and variability in the values.

The effectiveness of normalization will be impacted by the scale of the system being monitored. Shedding studies of normalizing agents PMMoV and CrAssphage demonstrate the wide range of shedding quantities among individuals (Arts et al., 2023). As a result, normalizing at small scales (e.g., less than 10,000) likely increases variability in the pathogen measurement (see Figure 4-2).

More studies are needed to understand the value of applying both viral and bacterial biomarkers as normalizing factors for the surveillance of different targets across a range of sewershed sizes, concentrations, and

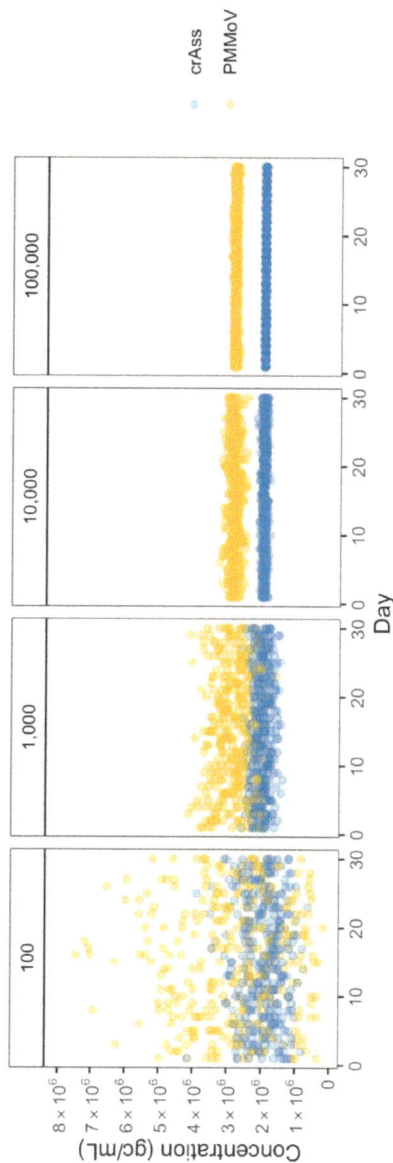

FIGURE 4-2 Predicted wastewater concentrations of two normalizing agents (crAssphage and PMMoV) in ideally mixed and perfectly composited samples from sewersheds containing between 100 and 100,000 people. Wastewater concentrations were generated from fecal shedding trajectories published in Arts et al. (2023).
SOURCE: Committee.

concentration/extraction methodologies. It is possible that one normalizing approach may work best for one pathogen/method/sewershed size, and another normalizing approach will work best for another pathogen/method/sewershed size. Candidate bacteria or viruses that are common to the human microbiome will have inherent biological variability within the sewershed population over time, and each may behave differently during transport due to differential partitioning to sediments and decay as they move through the system. For biomarkers associated with diet, different consumption rates between populations may complicate the comparisons of normalized values between sewersheds. Analyzing multiple constituents may initially be useful for understanding the sources of variability and could lead to development of a normalizing approach that considers multiple constituents.

The committee concluded that additional research using the large available data sets collected through the NWSS is needed to compare normalization methods across data from a range of different types of sites. Until coordinated and consistent normalization approaches are fully realized, non-normalized data should always be made available in NWSS for additional disease trend analysis.

VISUALIZATION AND DATA ANALYSIS TOOLS FOR INTEGRATION AND INTERPRETATION

The following section discusses the current state of data analysis and visualization tools for the NWSS, current challenges, and opportunities to better advance these systems to meet public health decision making. Both public-facing dashboards and analytical tools for public health agencies to assess trends and improve data integration are discussed. The committee recognizes that other data visualization platforms exist for subsets of the NWSS data (e.g., WastewaterSCAN,[2] Biobot Analytics[3]), but this section focuses on the NWSS as the largest data analysis and visualization platform in the United States that includes these other data.

Public-Facing Data Analysis and Visualization Tools

Jurisdiction-Level Tools

Currently, many states and localities that provide data to the NWSS have their own public-facing dashboard for data analysis and visualization. These dashboards were developed by state and local public health agencies

---

[2] See https://data.wastewaterscan.org/.
[3] See https://biobot.io/data/.

during the pandemic, at a time when CDC visualization tools were still developing, to meet their specific data visualization needs and the needs of the public and local decision makers outside the public health agency. As a result, the many independently developed state and local wastewater surveillance dashboards differ in how the magnitude, current trend direction, and time series of the virus are shown. These differences make aggregation or comparison across jurisdictions problematic and make it unclear to jurisdictions that are new to wastewater surveillance which method would best convey their information.

For example, with respect to COVID-19 wastewater surveillance, North Carolina, Virginia, and Wisconsin chose to represent and display the magnitude of viral load differently, making comparisons difficult (see Figure 4-3). Not only do the visual presentations vary, but descriptions of viral load levels are not easily comparable: Virginia and Wisconsin use words like "high" and "low," while North Carolina uses percentile ranges like "80-100%." North Carolina and Virginia do not state the exact time frame for their past samples, while Wisconsin's "past samples" are from the past 6 months.

Similarly, state and local dashboards differ in how trends of viral load are determined and conveyed, creating the same difficulties in comparing trends in viral loads geographically. Figure 4-4 illustrates such variation using the examples of Indiana, Utah, and Houston. All three dashboards use words like "increasing" and "decreasing" to describe the trend, but Houston includes four different rates of increase or decrease. The time frames represented in the data visualization also differ across the plots.

Finally, there are differences in how dashboards convey the viral load time series, again creating difficulty in comparisons and interpretations between areas. As shown in Figure 4-5, for example, the dashboards for New York, North Carolina, and Indiana differ in the extent to which individual sample data are emphasized over interpolations and the concentration presented (i.e., gene copies per person, gene copies per mL, and gene copies per human fecal marker PMMoV). For all three dashboard choices—virus intensity level, viral trends, and concentration versus time—differences in data presentation make comparisons more challenging.

A tool permitting the user to select their preference for data presentation to be displayed in one or more standard formats would allow for more options for interpretation and enable comparison between areas. Options for displaying the data in these three ways in a standard simple plug-and-play type of visualization and data analysis tool that jurisdictions can easily adopt would reduce the burden placed on public health agencies to develop and maintain individual dashboards. In a survey conducted by the Colorado and Houston NWSS Centers of Excellence, small public health agencies that serve fewer than one million people and public health agencies with less

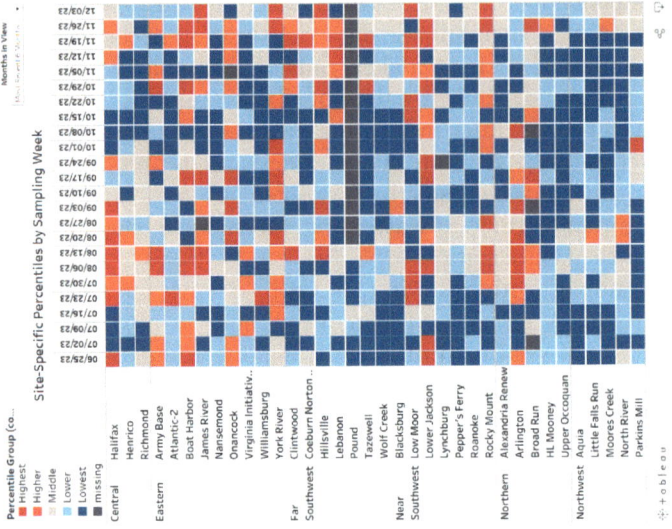

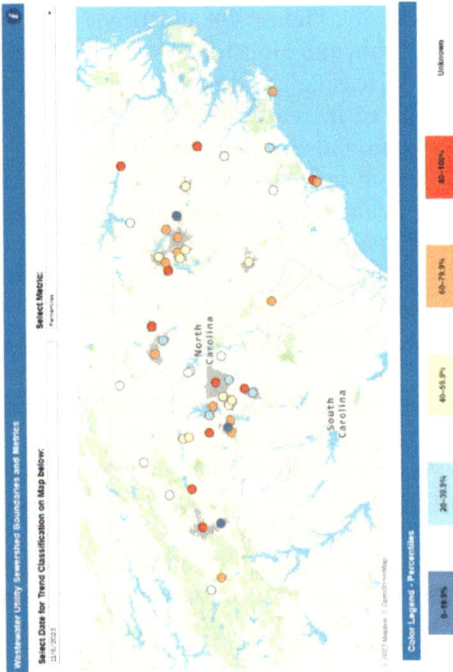

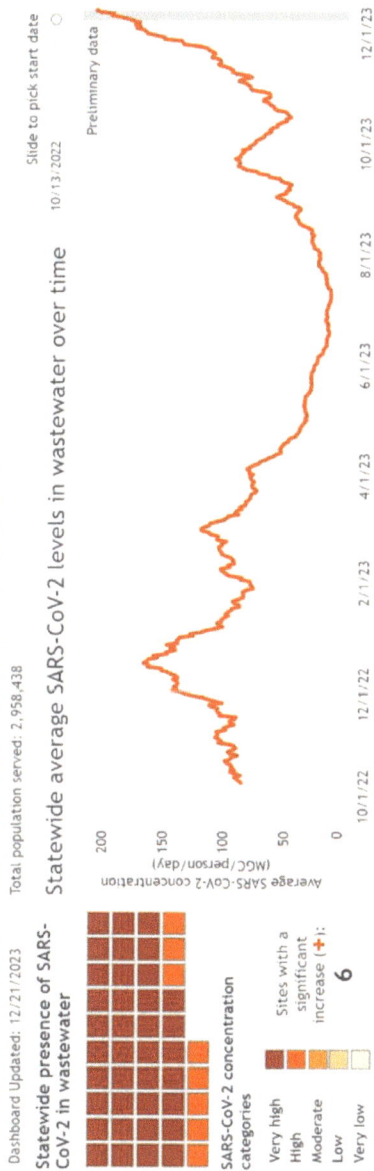

FIGURE 4-3 These three dashboard images provide examples of different and inconsistent methods used to indicate the magnitude of the wastewater viral load at a wastewater treatment plant. (a) North Carolina displays the magnitude as colored dots on a map with five categories, based on percentile of the current magnitude of the wastewater viral load relative to past conditions. (b) Virginia displays the metric of each location as a heatmap over time—not just the current data—and presents five categories ("Highest" to "Lowest," rather than exact percentile). The percentage breakdown is not readily apparent and so it cannot be compared to North Carolina. (c) Wisconsin displays the metric statewide, for each wastewater treatment plant, as a waffle chart ordered by magnitude in five categories using a different color scheme, and the category percentage breakdown is not readily apparent.
SOURCES: (a) https://covid19.ncdhhs.gov/dashboard/wastewater-monitoring; (b) https://www.vdh.virginia.gov/coronavirus/see-the-numbers/covid-19-data-insights/sars-cov-2-in-wastewater/; (c) https://www.dhs.wisconsin.gov/covid-19/wastewater.htm.

a)

b)

c)

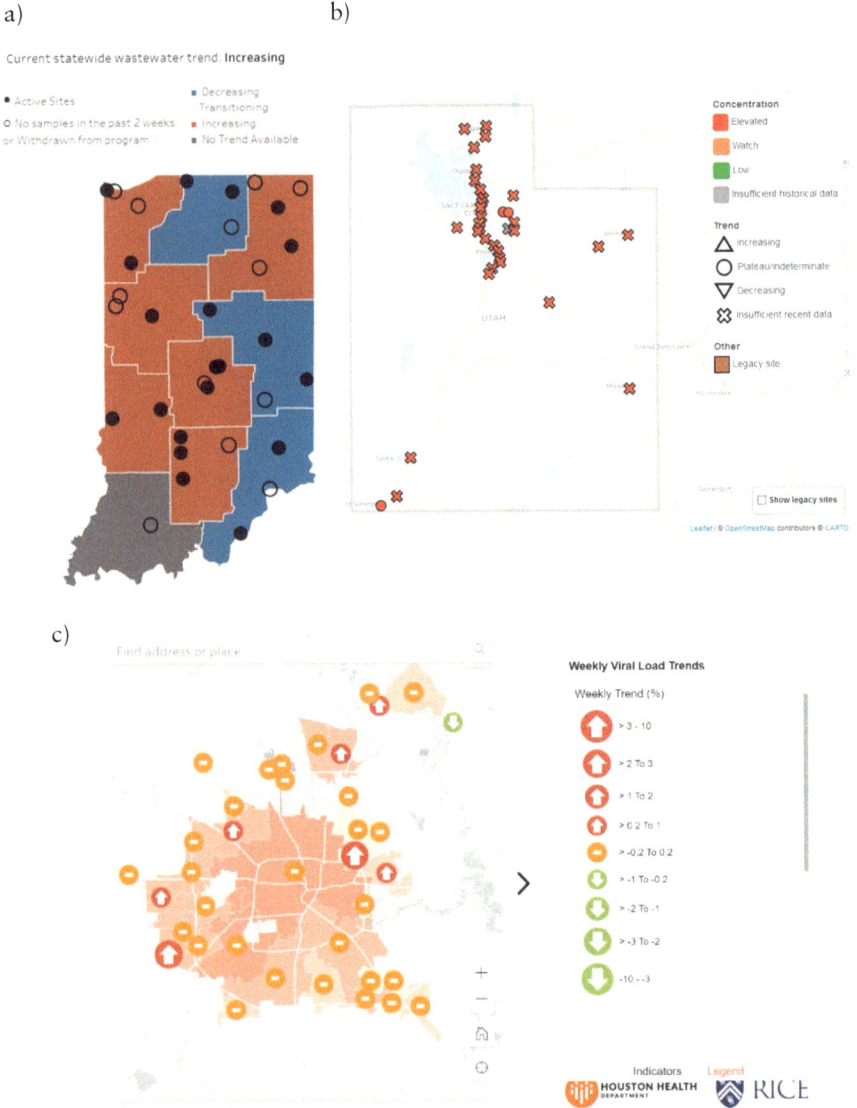

FIGURE 4-4 Three dashboard images showing different representations of wastewater viral load trends. (a) Indiana displays the trend in each of the state districts based on the wastewater treatment plant sampling sites in that district, (b) Utah displays the trend for each wastewater treatment plant via symbols on a map, and (c) Houston displays the trends as symbols on a map of the sewershed outlines. Indiana and Houston present trends based a 21-day window, while Utah's trend is based on the four most recent samples.

SOURCES: (a) https://www.coronavirus.in.gov/indiana-covid-19-dashboard-and-map/wastewater-dashboard/; (b) https://avrpublic.dhhs.utah.gov/uwss/; (c) https://covidwwtp.spatialstudieslab.org/.

75

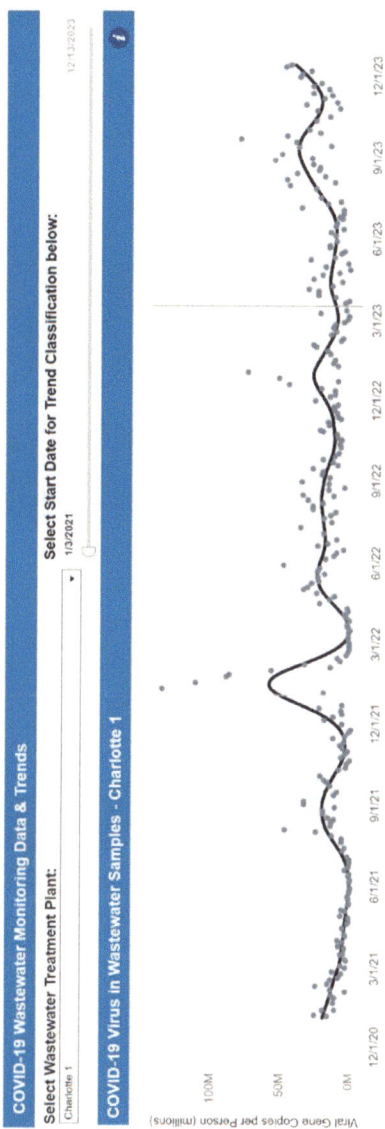

FIGURE 4-5 Three dashboard images with different representations of SARS-CoV-2 wastewater concentration results at a single site over time. (a) North Carolina displays individual sample concentrations along with spline estimates based on piecewise polynomial interpolation for data interpolation; (b) New York displays the raw wastewater concentration, with a symbol indicating if the result was above or below the detection limit; and (c) Indiana displays the smoothed wastewater concentration. North Carolina's wastewater concentration is the gene copies per person, New York's is the gene copies per mL, and Indiana's is the gene copies per human fecal marker pepper mild mottle virus (PMMoV).

SOURCES: (a) https://covid19.ncdhhs.gov/dashboard/wastewater-monitoring; (b) https://coronavirus.health.ny.gov/covid-19-waste-water-surveillance; (c) https://www.coronavirus.in.gov/indiana-covid-19-dashboard-and-map/wastewater-dashboard/.

continued

76

b)

c)

Statewide Wastewater Sample Concentration

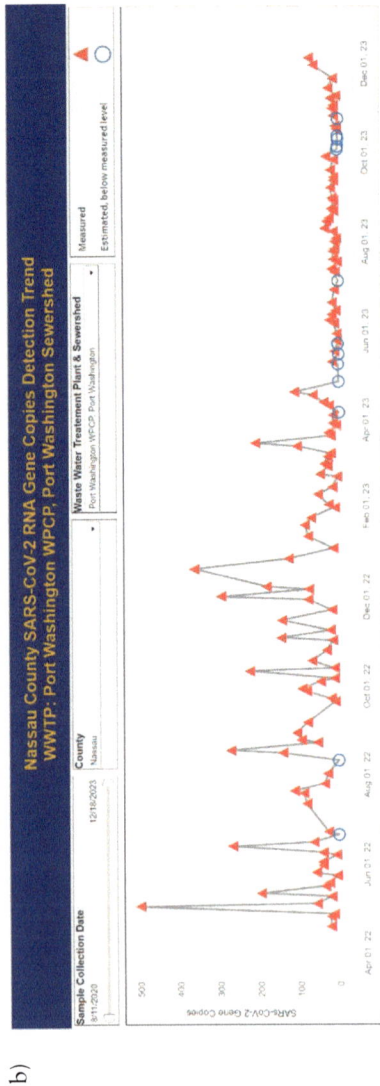

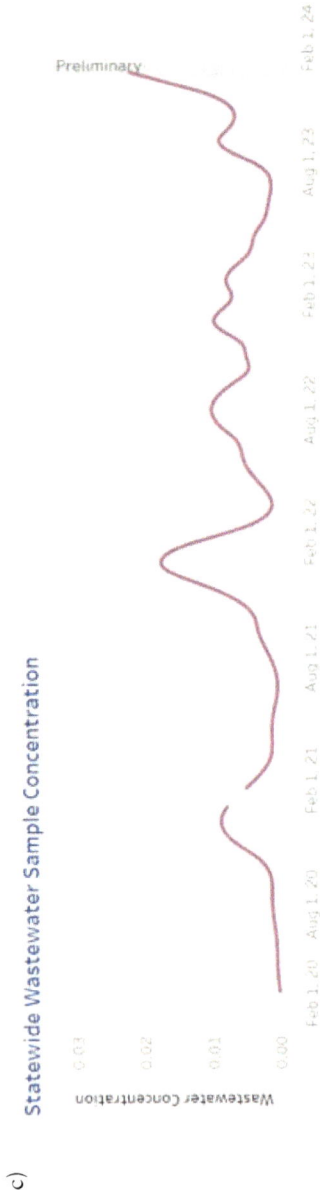

FIGURE 4-5 Continued

experience ranked developing a wastewater dashboard as the most important training need (R. Schneider, Houston Health Department and K. Weisbeck, Colorado Department of Health, personal communication, 2024).

NWSS Data Analysis and Visualization Tools:
COVID Data Tracker

CDC launched its own centralized data visualization of NWSS data on the COVID Data Tracker website in February 2022, targeted to the general public (Johnson, 2022). Until the NWSS data visualization tools were expanded in late 2023, the CDC dashboard (see Figure 4-6) primarily focused on a national map showing relative virus levels that were color-coded based on comparison to historical data at that site. Viewers could also see percentage change in the last 15 days (currently still available and based on a minimum of two data points). Due to a perceived risk of identifying particular sites, the NWSS dashboard currently only includes data from wastewater treatment plants serving over 3,000 people, and exact locations are not provided. Instead, each data point is plotted at the center of the ZIP code in which the wastewater treatment plant resides. This provides an easy-to-understand map of local areas of concern, but CDC acknowledges that the current viral-level data are not comparable across sites. The noncomparability arises from a wide range of factors, including that individual sites have been collecting data over different time periods. CDC notes on the website that the data history for sites that started reporting data after December 1, 2021, "is not long enough to reflect the same surges as the other sites."

Several notable enhancements have been recently added to the NWSS dashboard, including an additional dashboard for Mpox, SARS-CoV-2 variant data by site, and presentation of a new metric of viral activity (described in more detail below). A separate dashboard has been developed to summarize Mpox detection results over the last 4 weeks (see Figure 4-7). Users can adjust the view to get more information on states or individual sites; all data are plotted by ZIP code, to protect privacy.

Information on the temporal and spatial distribution of SARS-CoV-2 variants is now provided on a single webpage that presents data from nationally representative clinical samples from the National SARS-CoV-2 Genomic Surveillance System, clinical samples from arriving passengers at several major international airports via the Traveler-based SARS-CoV-2 Genomic Surveillance Program, and site-level wastewater surveillance.[4] The predominant variant is displayed graphically for each wastewater surveillance site based on the week selected by the user (see Figure 4-8a),

---

[4] See https://covid.cdc.gov/covid-data-tracker/#variant-summary.

and individual states can be selected to see how the relative abundance of variants has changed in that state over time (see Figure 4-8b). A separate page displays changes over time in the relative proportions of SARS-CoV-2 variants as national averages from wastewater data,[5] although the site notes that, because the sampling sites are not equally distributed across the nation, the data should not be considered a true national representation.

In addition to the map-based display of SARS-CoV-2 virus levels (Figure 4-4), the NWSS now displays a metric denoted the wastewater viral activity level (WVAL), which represents an aggregate of wastewater concentration data.[6] The NWSS provides weekly updates of national-, regional-, and state-level estimates of viral activity and trends over time (see Figure 4-9).[7] State-level data can be displayed graphically or in map form (Figure 4-10).

The WVAL metric was developed in an attempt to put different measures of viral levels into a common metric to improve national-, regional-, and state-level understanding of viral trends over time. A metric such as the WVAL would be very useful to track the virus at multiple scales. However, there are substantial weaknesses in the current WVAL metric and its use to track viral activity in time. The NWSS outlines four steps to calculate the WVAL, as described in Box 4-1. In the first step, data are adjusted via normalization based on data provided for each site. A weakness of this step is that data are carried through and aggregated, regardless of differences in normalization methods even though there is currently no scientific understanding of the differences in uncertainty introduced between the two normalization methods. Without adjustment for these differences, the WVAL metric will be influenced by the uncertainty and percentage of sites normalized differently. Further research is needed to correctly account for the uncertainty introduced when combining data normalized differently and whether normalization is beneficial to the assessment of disease burden across multiple locations.

In the second step, "for each combination of site, data submitter, PCR target, laboratory methods, and normalization method," a baseline is calculated. A weakness of the second step is that whenever any of these factors changes, the baseline is reset. When sites have less than 12 months of data, the baseline risks missing annual temporal patterns. For example, a 3-month baseline that includes peak RSV levels would not be useful to pick up a peak that occurs in the next 6 months because it would not appear high. Once the baseline is 12 months long, this systematic baseline selection weakness may not be as much of a concern, but research should be conducted to inform the decision whether to require a minimum of 12

---

[5] See https://www.cdc.gov/nwss/rv/COVID19-variants.html.
[6] See https://covid.cdc.gov/covid-data-tracker/#wastewater-surveillance.
[7] See https://www.cdc.gov/nwss/rv/COVID19-nationaltrend.html.

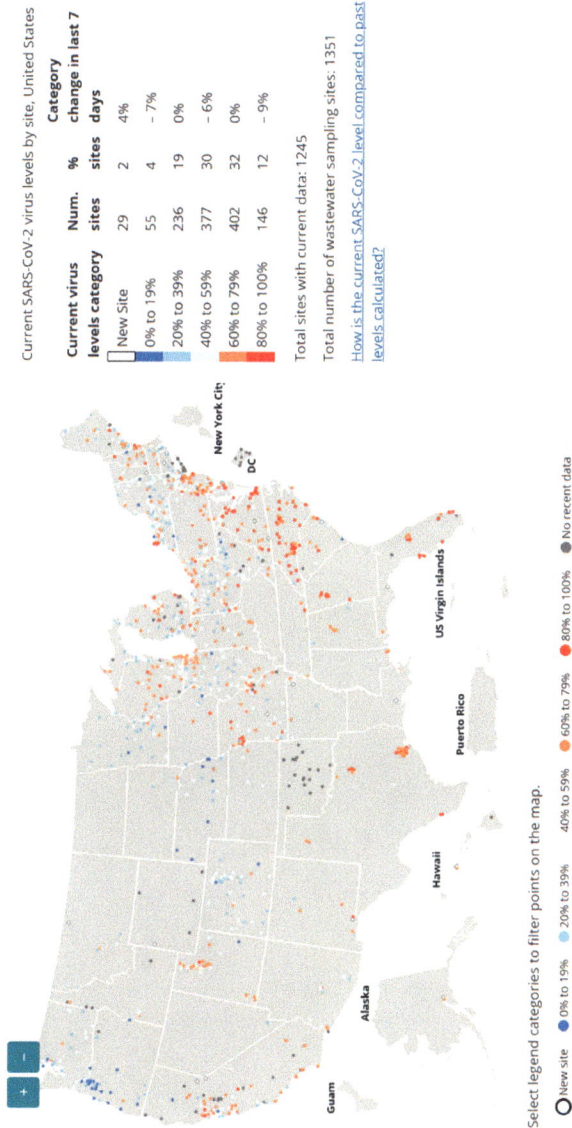

Current SARS-CoV-2 virus levels by site, United States

Current virus levels category	Num. sites	% sites	Category change in last 7 days
New Site	29	2	4%
0% to 19%	55	4	- 7%
20% to 39%	236	19	0%
40% to 59%	377	30	- 6%
60% to 79%	402	32	0%
80% to 100%	146	12	- 9%

Total sites with current data: 1245

Total number of wastewater sampling sites: 1351

How is the current SARS-CoV-2 level compared to past levels calculated?

Select legend categories to filter points on the map.

○ New site ● 0% to 19% ● 20% to 39% ● 40% to 59% ● 60% to 79% ● 80% to 100% ● No recent data

FIGURE 4-6 NWSS wastewater metric map showing current SARS-CoV-2 virus levels by site on February 26, 2024, relative to the historical data.
SOURCE: https://covid.cdc.gov/covid-data-tracker/#wastewater-surveillance.

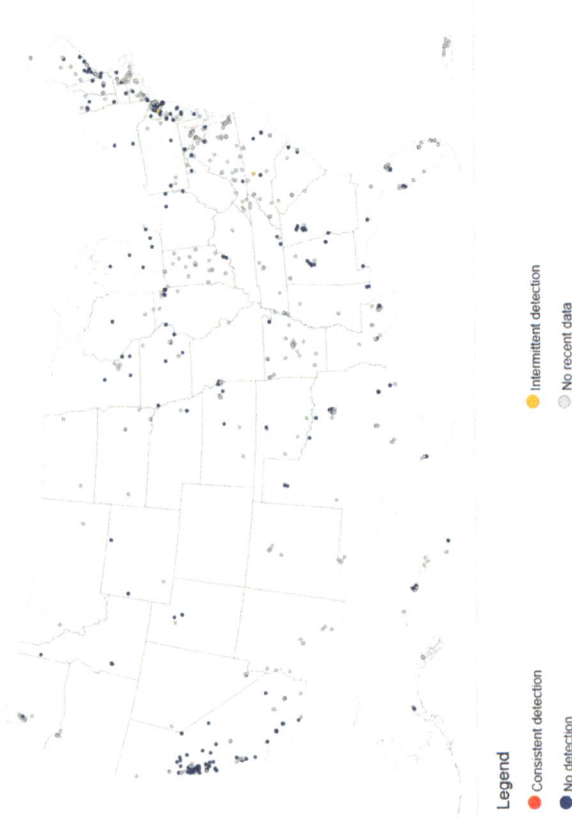

FIGURE 4-7 Dashboard showing Mpox virus detection over the previous 4 weeks. The data are plotted based on the ZIP code of the sampling location. Consistent detection is described as where Mpox virus was detected in more than 80% of samples in the past 4 weeks and the most recent detection was within the past 2 weeks. Intermittent detection is where Mpox virus was detected in 1% to 80% of samples in the past 4 weeks and the most recent detection was within the past 2 weeks.
SOURCE: https://www.cdc.gov/nwss/wastewater-surveillance/mpox-data.html (accessed February 27, 2024).

months of baseline data for the WVAL metric. Additionally, no mention is made of whether (or how) nondetections are used in the computation of the baseline or the standard deviation. The use of the standard deviation over a nonparametric measure of spread (e.g., the interquartile range divided by 4) requires consideration of the nondetection values, but the method for calculating the standard deviation is not discussed.

In the third step of the WVAL, a WVAL for each sample from a site is calculated and then the mean WVAL for a week is calculated for the site. A weakness of the third step is again around the eventual aggregation of values with different levels of uncertainty. The use of the weekly averaged values allows for sites that have only one value to be aggregated alongside averages from sites with multiple weekly values, the latter of which will be smoother. Consideration should be given to using a fixed number of samples from each site each week for comparison to the standard deviation. Also, not all sites or measurements from a given site are used (e.g., if a site is measured by WastewaterSCAN as well as by local jurisdictions), and it is not always clear to localities which sites are represented by the WVAL metric or why.

Overall, there are two additional weaknesses of the WVAL four-step approach (see Box 4-1). First, the standard deviation is used to put all the site data, which are collected in different ways and normalized by different means, on the same scale so that they can be aggregated and compared. The problem is that the variation in the magnitudes of standard deviations due to the disease burden in a community is not reflected. For example, a site with a highly variable viral load due to fluctuating disease burden will have a large standard deviation in its WVAL calculation, and a second site with very little virus (i.e., near the detection limit) would have a relatively constant viral load with a very small standard deviation in its WVAL calculation. The weekly concentration at each site could end up being the same number of standard deviations away from the baseline, resulting in the same WVAL, although the first site clearly has more virus and merits different responses. Thus, the use of the WVAL to make statements about the overall viral load across the United States triggered by an increase in standard deviation could be misleading. Second, the aggregation does not account for the unequal distribution of sites across the nation, region, or state. For example, because over 50 percent of the WVAL data for Texas are generated in Houston, the state's viral load will most likely be from Houston, although it is presented as a figure for the entire state (see Figure 4-10).

Presenting a global metric is important to enable comparisons across sites, but additional work is needed to address existing limitations and improve the scientific basis for the calculations. As NWSS continues to refine the WVAL, it should also stay abreast of other efforts, such as by WastewaterSCAN (see Box 4-2), to develop similar aggregation and comparison

82

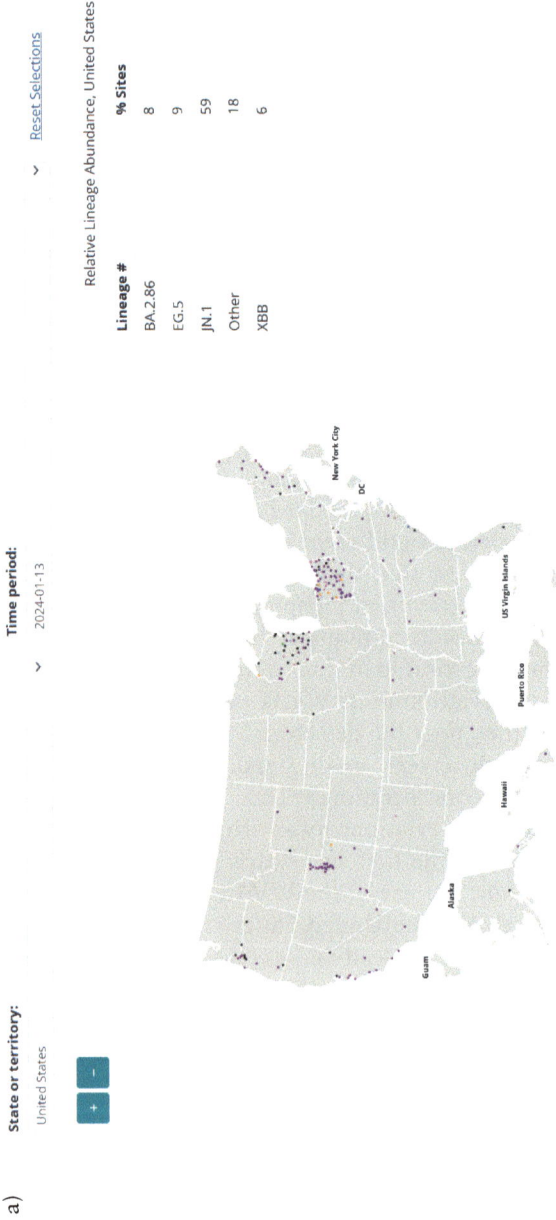

FIGURE 4-8 Images from the CDC website summary of variant surveillance showing variant data by sampling site at (a) a national level for a specified week and (b) at a state level, where recent trends are plotted.
SOURCE: https://covid.cdc.gov/covid-data-tracker/#variant-summary (accessed February 27, 2024).

FIGURE 4-8 Continued

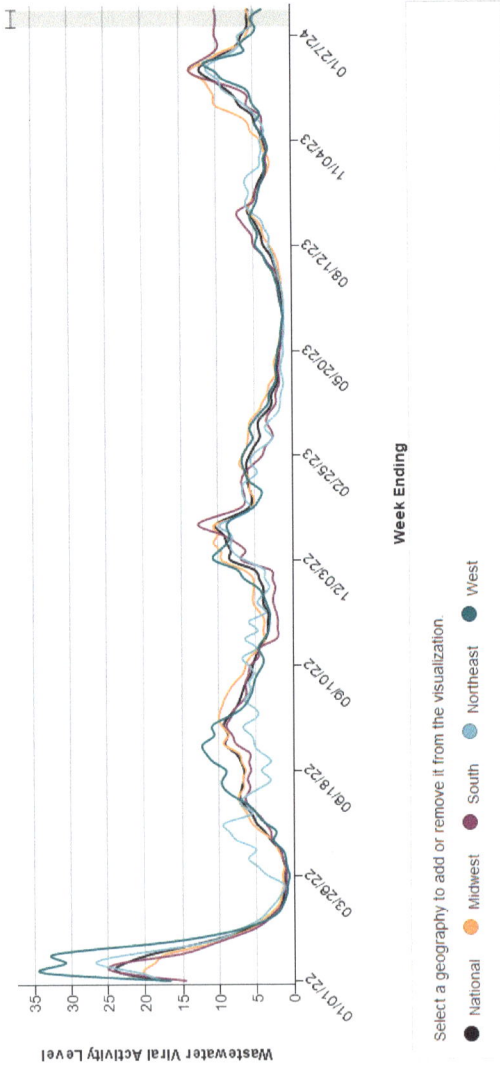

FIGURE 4-9 National and regional trends of SARS-CoV-2 viral activity levels in wastewater. The gray shading represents the most recent 2-week period in which the data may be incomplete due to delays in data reporting.
SOURCE: https://www.cdc.gov/nwss/rv/COVID19-nationaltrend.html (accessed February 27, 2024).

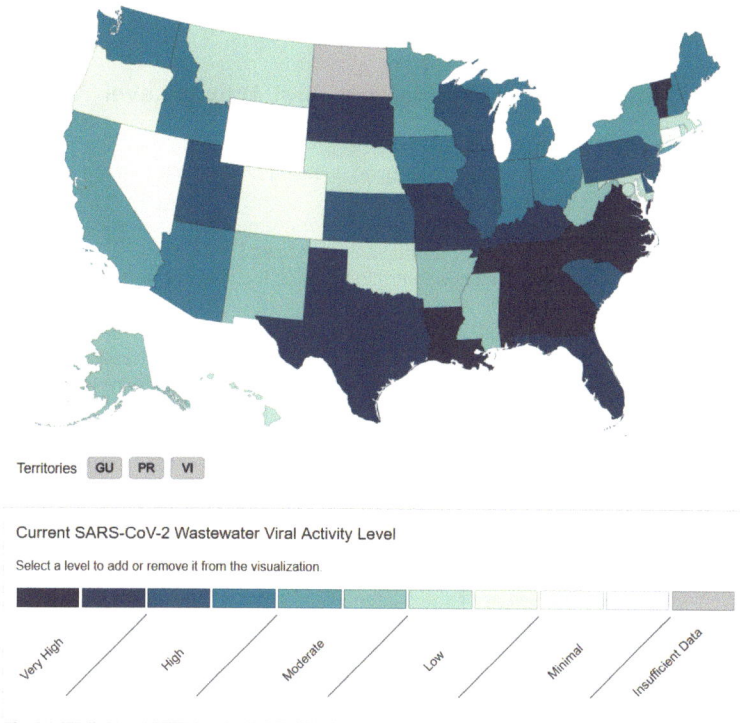

FIGURE 4-10 Map showing SARS-CoV-2 viral activity levels by state.
SOURCE: https://www.cdc.gov/nwss/rv/COVID19-currentlevels.html (accessed February 27, 2024).

metrics and their comparative successes and limitations. A large-scale analysis of the most successful wastewater surveillance metrics could evaluate the extent to which these metrics are concordant or discordant when fed the same data, and which metrics are most predictive or correlated with clinical data (e.g., hospitalizations). More extensive research is needed to compare a wide range of alternative approaches to spatial aggregation (using different pathogens, time periods, and methods), to explore how different methods and models can be used to generate consistent aggregate statistics.

Looking Ahead

Advancing trend analyses. Currently, public-facing dashboards in the NWSS do not evaluate or label the trend in loads (e.g., increasing, decreasing) or provide forecasts, and individual jurisdictions employ different

BOX 4-1
Calculating the Wastewater Viral Activity Level

1. **Data Normalization:**
   - The type of data normalization used is based on the data that are submitted by the site.
     - □ If both flow-population and microbial normalization values are available, flow-population normalization is used.
   - After normalization, all concentration data is log transformed.

2. **Baseline Calculation:**
   - For each combination of site, data submitter, PCR target, lab methods, and normalization method, a baseline is established. The "baseline" is the 10th percentile of the log-transformed and normalized concentration data within a specific time frame.
     - □ For site and method combinations (as listed above) with over 6 months of data, baselines are re-calculated every six calendar months (January 1 and July 1) using the past 12 months of data.
     - □ For sites and method combinations with less than six months of data, baselines are computed weekly until reaching six months, after which they remain unchanged until the next January 1 or July 1, at which time baselines are recalculated.
   - The standard deviation for each site and method combination is calculated using the same time frame as the baseline.

3. **Wastewater Viral Activity Level Calculation:**
   - The number of standard deviations that each log-transformed concentration value deviates from the baseline (positive if above, negative if below) is calculated.
   - This value (x) is then converted back to a linear scale (by calculating e^x) to form the Wastewater Viral Activity Level for the site and method combination.
   - The Wastewater Viral Activity Levels from a site are averaged by week for all figures.

4. **Aggregation for National, Regional, and State Levels:**
   - We calculate the median Wastewater Viral Activity Levels among sites at national, regional, and state levels, excluding data from site/method combinations with less than 6 weeks of data.

Data Inclusion Criteria: New NWSS wastewater sampling sites, or sites with a substantial change in laboratory methods are included in national, regional, state, or territorial median values once there are at least 6 weeks of samples reported for that location. States or territories without sufficient data to estimate the wastewater viral activity level for the previous week are indicated as "Insufficient Data."

SOURCE: https://www.cdc.gov/nwss/about-data.html#data-method.

BOX 4-2
WastewaterSCAN Aggregation Metric

WastewaterSCAN also provides a national dashboard with aggregation metrics at the county, state, regional, and national levels. In the SCAN case, aggregated trend lines and levels are calculated using the trimmed smoothed average PMMoV-normalized concentration for each site, multiplied by the catchment area population, and then divided by the overall region population, to yield a weighted average of normalized concentration over n plants within a region:

$$Aggregated\ Target\ Level = \frac{\sum_{i=1}^{n} pop_i \cdot trimmed\, \frac{Target}{PMMoV_i}}{\sum_{i=1}^{n} pop_i}$$

Nondetections are set to approximately half of the limit of detection for the purposes of this calculation. Regional and national trend lines and levels are calculated in a similar fashion, but with states as the averaged unit rather than individual treatment plants. Levels for these aggregated regions are set using tertiles of the historical distribution over the past 365 days to reflect a low/medium/high range for each pathogen target and region.

An advantage of SCAN in the calculation of aggregated trends and levels is that the SCAN data use the same measurement and normalization approaches for all of their samples, which facilitates ease of comparison. However, this approach has its limitations as well. Using the past 365 days to generate the historical distribution means that the low/medium/high level ranges may potentially change day to day, which can hinder easy or consistent interpretability and potentially make the same concentration at a given site imply a different level depending on when it occurs. Either a longer time window to smooth across multiple years, or a fixed level update schedule (e.g., annually or every n years) might improve interpretability. Additionally, while using percentile ranks/tertiles is straightforward and interpretable as low/medium/high, different sites may have different histories as far as the level of outbreak/transmission they have experienced, potentially leading to artificially condensed level ranges if a given site simply has not experienced as extensive of an epidemic as another.

SOURCE: https://data.wastewaterscan.org/about/ (accessed July 6, 2024).

statistical methods to analyze trends.[8] Moving forward it is important to develop statistical strategies that separate the signal or trend of disease burden as measured by wastewater from the inherent sampling and measurement variation associated with each sample. To develop these tools for application at a national scale, research is needed to understand which techniques work best overall and the implications of factors that vary by jurisdiction (e.g., sampling frequency, population coverage, percent of nondetections). As a simple example, rolling averages are most commonly used currently to evaluate a basic visual trend, but these may not be the most appropriate smoothing method for wastewater data; further research to evaluate which trend methods best balance simplicity and flexibility for wastewater data would be a strong first step. The most appropriate statistical methods may vary based upon the wastewater target. For example, in scenarios where there are very high frequencies of nondetections (as will likely be more common as the targets are expanded beyond SARS-CoV-2), methods that are better at handling censored data will need to be employed, and within this subset, these methods may differ depending upon the rarity of detects. The uncertainty around the trend line should accompany the graph and incorporate temporal dependencies of the data.

To accomplish this research, available wastewater surveillance data across the nation will need to be analyzed using a range of statistical trend and forecasting methods. Researchers need access to all the historical wastewater data including detection limits, sampling method and frequency, treatment plant population coverage, and laboratory analytical methods. In this analysis, it is also important to incorporate the inherent sampling and laboratory variability for each location sample.

Advancing a common platform for the public. A common platform providing analytics that assess trend, define the viral load, and explain the inference in language that is understandable to the lay public would be a more effective communication tool than maintaining distinctive dashboards for each jurisdiction, and would also reduce burden on local health agencies. The greater standardization in presentation that a centralized platform would bring would also improve interpretation and comparability across jurisdictions, facilitate aggregation, and promote communication across stakeholders. However, care needs to be taken in the extent and method of

---

[8] For example, Wisconsin uses a linear regression over the past five measurements with a relaxed significance test (p < 0.3), Illinois uses a locally weighted scatterplot smoothing method, North Carolina uses a spline, and Missouri uses an exponentially weighted moving average. Of these examples, only Illinois provides confidence intervals around the trendline. SOURCES: https://www.dhs.wisconsin.gov/covid-19/wastewater.htm; https://iwss.uillinois.edu/wastewater-treatment-plants/, https://iwss.uillinois.edu/; https://covid19.ncdhhs.gov/dashboard/wastewater-monitoring; and https://storymaps.arcgis.com/stories/f7f5492486114da6b5d6fdc07f81aacf.

aggregation so that the interpretation is scientifically correct. For example, in Houston, the 39 wastewater treatment plants represent a total population of 2.2 million people but plants vary in size, covering a range of 600 to over 550,000 people. Pooled analyses that do not use weighting to account for this variation in representation may generate misleading information.

Through the pandemic, some members of the public and the press became educated on what wastewater surveillance was and what it meant to them, often through multiple interactions between health departments and the media. With the advent of a common visualization tool with consistent reporting, the burden of interpretation can be met by CDC or the Centers of Excellence, as needed.

The dashboard's public-facing language should also be made available in languages other than English to promote equity of access to information. Currently, no dashboards are available in other languages, although Colorado does have a Spanish version of its dashboard FAQ file. This results in some notable exclusions of non-English-speaking populations from the benefits of publicly shared wastewater data. For example, the dashboard in Houston, Texas, is English only, although about 15 percent of households in the City of Houston have limited English proficiency.

Tools for Public Health Agencies

DCIPHER

The NWSS currently offers data analysis and visualization tools within the Data Collation and Integration for Public Health Event Response (DCIPHER) platform. DCIPHER "is a cloud-based data integration and management platform for use across CDC, in the Emergency Operations Center, by other federal partners, and by state, local, tribal, and territorial public health jurisdictions to collate, link, manage, analyze, visualize, and share public health, outbreak, and event response data" (HHS, 2020). Analytical laboratories upload their results and associated metadata to DCIPHER, and the platform includes data quality checks and alerts. DCIPHER also includes resources for NWSS jurisdictions, including guidance documents, training materials, and points of contact to promote peer-to-peer collaboration. The content of DCIPHER is not publicly available, and only the jurisdiction that submits data to DCIPHER can download those data.

Within DCIPHER, Contour—a program developed by a third party—provides a method to join data sets and explore trends, percentiles, and other graphics in a point-and-click format. The types of analyses available in Contour are useful (e.g., flow-population normalized trend with interpretation of sustained decrease, decrease, plateau, increase, and sustained increase; percent change; proportion detected; comparisons of percentages in a region). However, some individual jurisdictions are currently employing statistical analyses not available as plug-and-play tools in Contour (e.g., Figure 4-5), and CDC is currently working to develop additional tools (H. Reese, CDC, personal communication, 2023). Jurisdictions can write code (termed "paths") to replicate the analyses from week to week, although this requires training for those unfamiliar with coding. Although the NWSS provides training videos to help users with Contour, large public health agencies still ranked trainings centered around analyzing data for trends as their most important training need (R. Schneider, Houston Health Department and K. Weisbeck, Colorado Department of Health, personal communication, 2024). In general, a tool developed in a more versatile broadly applied language (e.g., R) instead of niche software would make training more efficient.

In addition, there are sometimes errors in the analysis and interpretation in DCIPHER's NWSS and Improved Dashboard; or if there are underlying statistical reasons for these interpretations, they are not explained to the user. For example, Figure 4-11 displays the analysis for a small site in Texas (Laredo), with a spline fit showing a peak in late August and an interpretation that the data are plateaued (yellow bar) from the end of July to September. The graph and the interpretation are inconsistent, and no explanation is provided. Similarly, the interpretation for a large facility in Houston indicates that the flow-population normalized trend is a sustained decrease from the middle of April 2022 to the middle of April 2023 while the spline fit shows two distinct peaks during that period (see Figure 4-12). As a third example, flow is not reported for some sites but Contour provides flow-normalized trends.

In general, problems with data interpretation and the steep learning curve have led to concerns using DCIPHER/Contour for data analysis, and large jurisdictions and public health authorities generally continue to use their own analytical tools, which limits their capacity to understand their data in a broader context. Currently, Contour is best suited for exploring data in different ways using simple methods, but not in-depth analyses. Additionally, Contour is not appropriate for those that are not familiar with analysis of wastewater surveillance data due to its sometimes inconsistent interpretations (as shown in Figures 4-11 and 4-12).

Advancing Statistical Tools in Collaboration with
Local or State Jurisdictions

Ultimately, local, state, and national public health agencies need data analysis tools that are reliable, easy to use, and able to accommodate the specific characteristics and analysis needs of individual jurisdictions. The committee recognizes that there are many constraints on the use of

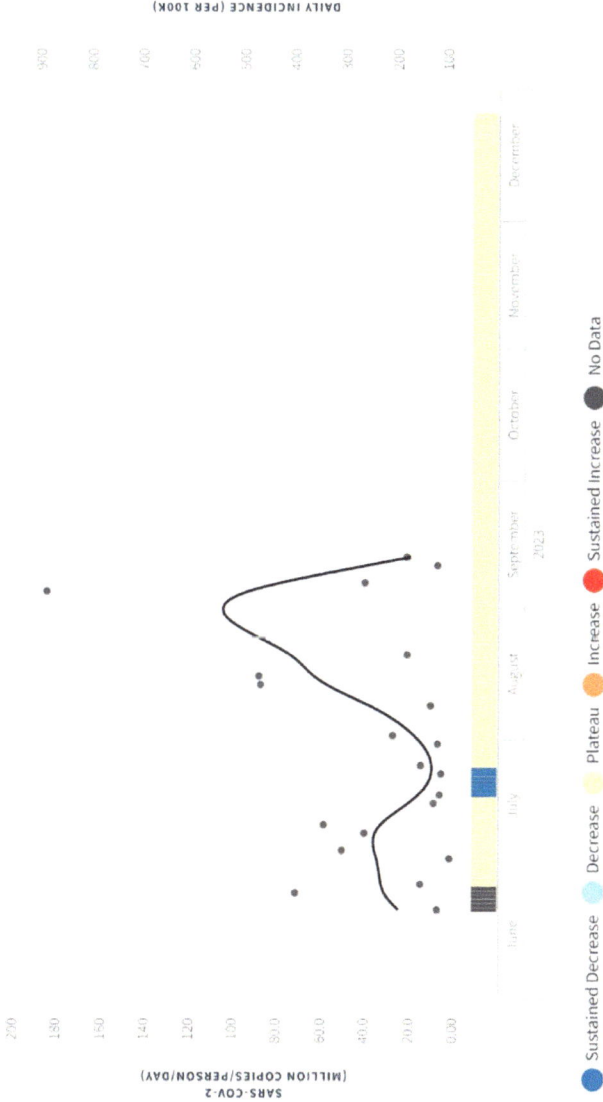

FIGURE 4-11 SARS-CoV-2 levels in wastewater in Laredo, Texas, as analyzed by DCIPHER. The line represents a spline fit, which is a type of regression methodology. The interpretation of decrease versus plateau seems inconsistent with the data.
SOURCE: NWSS and Improved Dashboard (accessed December 26, 2023).

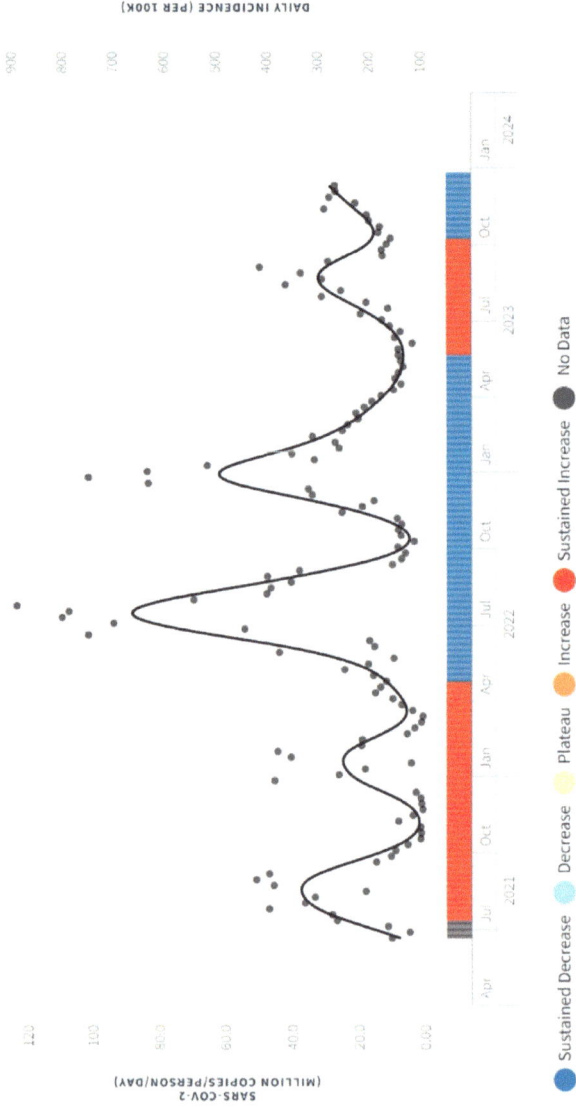

FIGURE 4-12 SARS-CoV-2 levels from a wastewater treatment plant in Houston, Texas, as analyzed by DCIPHER. The interpretation of sustained decrease versus sustained increase (see blue and red bar below the plotted data) seems inconsistent with the data.
SOURCE: NWSS and Improved Dashboard (accessed December 26, 2023).

DCIPHER, which has applications far beyond wastewater surveillance data, including data security requirements that may make code revisions cumbersome and limit those who are allowed to access DCIPHER.

Until CDC develops easy-to-use analytical tools that meet the needs of local and state jurisdictions, code sharing would help jurisdictions that are just starting their wastewater surveillance program advance their data analytics at a faster rate. CDC could use DCIPHER for centralized data storage and access, with standardized metadata, and use those data to populate the public-facing dashboards. Jurisdictions could easily download the interoperable data for additional analyses with shared, open-access code.

Currently, some large and sophisticated public health agencies are advancing tools to assess and forecast trends. These jurisdictions could work collaboratively with CDC, other federal agencies, and the Centers of Excellence to build on the existing understanding of the best methods to statistically interpret wastewater data. To advance such an effort, code and data sharing in a publicly accessible location (e.g., GitHub) would be valuable for researchers and jurisdictions. A common language (or two) for analysis should also be selected. Previous NWSS meetings suggest this would be R, although a formal survey should be conducted. The NWSS Centers of Excellence can assist with training and building out the dashboards so that areas without this specific expertise are provided the needed support. During this interim period, each jurisdiction would be the owner of their own sample code and data. Code and data sharing has not yet taken place in a meaningful way in the NWSS community. Houston has created a Github with two repositories,[9] and some states, like New York,[10] have made their wastewater data but not their code publicly available.

Improving Tools for Clinical Data Integration

As noted in the committee's Phase 1 report (NASEM, 2023), rigorous interpretation of wastewater surveillance requires integration with clinical data, where available and reliable. A visualization tool that automatically displays cases from reportable disease systems and/or syndromic systems, along with immunization rates within and around the jurisdiction for easy comparison with wastewater viral loads across time for each specific target, would be useful. When a wastewater target is not detected and no cases are detected, the surveillance provides a level of reassurance. When a wastewater target is detected before clinical cases are found, the public health team can initiate the wastewater response action plan as needed. When clinical cases are detected in the sewershed prior to detection in wastewater, the

---

[9] See https://github.com/hou-wastewater-epi-org.
[10] See https://coronavirus.health.ny.gov/covid-19-wastewater-surveillance.

wastewater team may need to evaluate the sampling and analysis strategy relative to the overall goals, and determine whether additional refinements of the sampling strategy, re-analysis of prior samples, or lower detection limits are needed. Constant comparisons between wastewater and clinical data may identify potential problems in one approach or the other. Advancements in machine learning could provide more comprehensive understanding of public health dynamics and improve public health responses.

The committee recognizes that integration of wastewater data with clinical data systems, such as emergency department syndromic surveillance systems, reportable diseases systems, and vaccine tracking systems, is a major challenge because the clinical data systems themselves are not integrated. It should also be noted that clinical data can be disparate, incomplete, and not representative for many important diseases. However, improved and integrated data systems would support more informed rapid response to infectious disease outbreaks.

Emergency department syndromic surveillance data. Emergency department (ED) syndromic surveillance systems provide constant monitoring of trends in counts of individuals with severe illness by syndrome (e.g., respiratory, gastrointestinal illness) visiting EDs or urgent care centers based on symptoms, chief complaints, and discharge diagnosis. These data are anonymized, including only the patient age and ZIP code. Like wastewater surveillance viral load information, the ED syndromic data are used to provide a measure of illness by geographic unit. Stable trends provide reassurance when an impact has not occurred while increases provide notice of early warning of an outbreak. This surveillance is timelier than the reportable disease system, which requires laboratory test results. Also, because syndromes are more flexible and generally defined, syndromic surveillance is better poised to pick up emerging outbreaks (Hughes et al., 2020).

The evolution of the development and use of wastewater surveillance data in public health is similar to that which occurred in ED syndromic surveillance in that the national system was built upon pre-existing local systems that were then expanded (Hughes et al., 2020). Similar obstacles need to be overcome in cross-jurisdiction use of ED syndromic surveillance as with cross-jurisdiction analysis of wastewater surveillance, including the need for unified metrics, consistent statistical interpretation, mapping, and timeliness. Current local ED syndromic surveillance systems in the United States (i.e., Electronic Surveillance System for the Early Notification of Community-Based Epidemics [ESSENCE]) use unified queries and feed into the U.S. National Syndromic Surveillance Program (NSSP). Considering this history, best practices and lessons from merging the local ED syndromic systems into the national system, such as the need to report and interpret the data in aggregate to improve public health response, should be applied to the national wastewater surveillance system.

During the COVID-19 pandemic, a few individual jurisdictions developed data visualizations to display the wastewater surveillance viral load alongside other clinical data, including ED syndromic data (e.g., Figure 4-13). At the Houston Health Department, to integrate the wastewater data with the syndromic data from ESSENCE, the wastewater data are shared with the syndromic team and plotted together. The data sharing and plotting is not automated and requires cooperation between groups that may not be in the same departments in a jurisdiction.

Instead of each jurisdiction integrating their wastewater viral load data alongside the area ED syndromic data, an automatic mapping of these data back to the jurisdiction from NSSP would be more efficient. This would be especially helpful for smaller jurisdictions without the workforce capacity to routinely map the data. Numbers of visits linked to specific International Classification of Diseases codes or respiratory or gastrointestinal syndromic data could be displayed as per pertinence to the wastewater target of interest. If the jurisdiction does not report to an ESSENCE system, NSSP could provide information from surrounding areas.

Reportable disease system data. Reportable disease system platforms record cases by statutory requirement. CDC requires some specific diseases to be reported but the total list can vary by state. The information on confirmed or suspected cases in this system lags information from ED syndromic surveillance and does not include some diseases of specific interest in wastewater (e.g., influenza A/B or RSV), but it includes more specific information (i.e., patient/illness details that inform case follow-up and tracking).

During the COVID-19 pandemic, some jurisdictions with both wastewater surveillance systems and reportable disease systems incorporated case counts obtained from their reportable disease systems in time series of wastewater viral load to aid in interpretation of trends (see Figure 4-14). Going forward, routine incorporation of case data alongside wastewater viral load data for specific diseases that are measured in the wastewater and reportable would be extremely helpful.

Locally hosted reportable disease systems report their data to their state health department, which then reports to the CDC National Notifiable Diseases Surveillance System (NNDSS).[11] The NNDSS system and those reporting to it (i.e., all 50 states) are based on the National Electronic Disease Surveillance System architectural standards to ensure interoperability between systems.[12] Assuming NDSS data quality and reporting turnaround

---

[11] See https://www.cdc.gov/nndss/index.html.
[12] See https://www.cdc.gov/nndss/about/nedss.html.

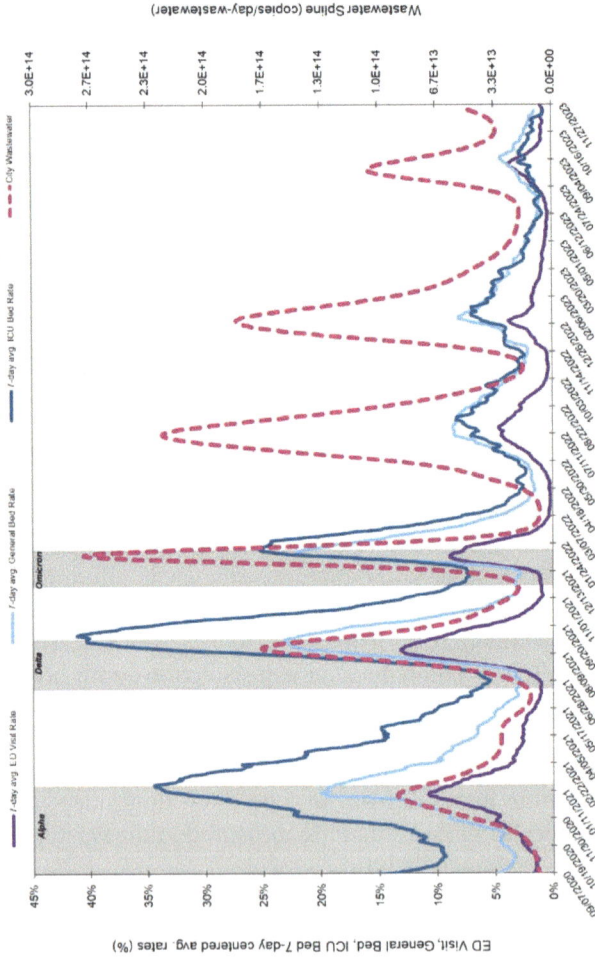

FIGURE 4-13 The Houston Health Department combines data sets to plot 7-day averages of emergency department (ED) visits, hospital bed use, and intensive care unit (ICU) bed use alongside wastewater surveillance viral levels. SOURCE: Hopkins et al., 2023.

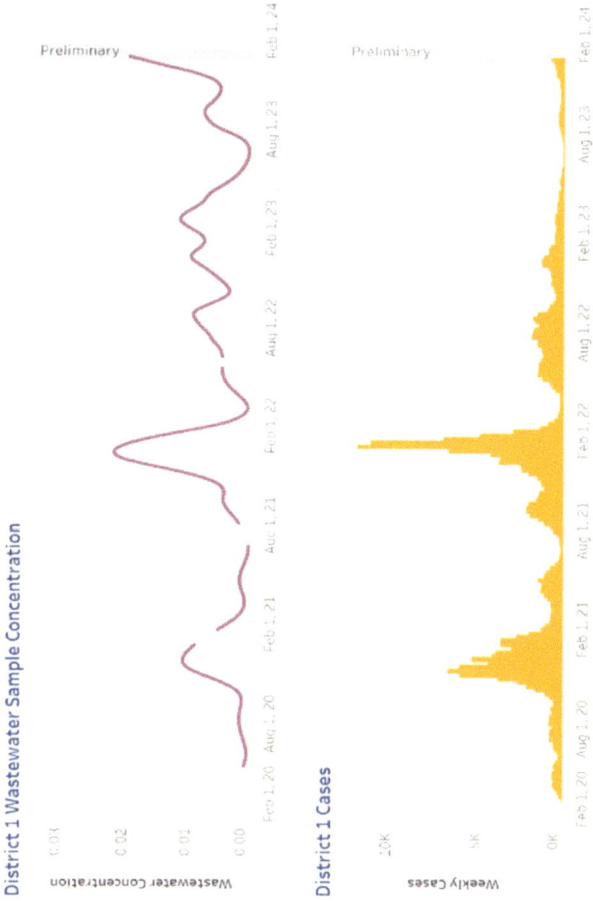

FIGURE 4-14 Indiana's COVID-19 dashboard presents the count of weekly new positive cases against SARS-CoV-2 concentration in wastewater data.

SOURCE: https://www.coronavirus.in.gov/indiana-covid-19-dashboard-and-map/wastewater-dashboard/.

times are reasonable, an automatic mapping of these data back to the jurisdiction from NNDSS would be more efficient and especially helpful for smaller jurisdictions that may not have reportable cases in their jurisdiction but would benefit from the knowledge of the extent of area cases.

Immunization data. Immunization database systems that provide rates of immunizations by geographic unit (e.g., census tract or ZIP code) by type, gender, and age group were found to be important for understanding vaccine uptake and targeting interventions during the COVID-19 pandemic. Integrating wastewater viral load and vaccination rate information for vaccine-preventable diseases from the CDC Immunization Information System[13] would provide important information for local health departments. Data should include not just required vaccines but others, such as influenza and RSV. For example, when influenza is found to be increasing in wastewater, influenza vaccine events can be directed to areas where uptake is low or, as mentioned previously, vaccination information can inform the frequency of monitoring for a specific target (i.e., high vaccination rates may trigger reduced surveillance).

Improving Timeliness of Wastewater Data

Wastewater data, like many other data systems, can suffer from a range of delays associated with the transport of samples, analytical processing, and data reporting. These delays can erode the time in which the data can inform public health decision making and potentially the impacts of those decisions. As discussed in Chapter 2, sampling frequency also affects the timeliness of information provided, particularly in terms of evaluating changes in trends. In many cases, if the most recent wastewater data available are more than 1 to 2 weeks old, it may not provide actionable information that can practically inform decision making, as the situation on the ground may have changed since the sample was collected.

In a recent analysis of the timeliness of wastewater data posted by several wastewater surveillance programs, there were sizable differences between programs (see Figure 4-15; J. Gilbert and M. Eisenberg, University of Michigan, personal communication, 2024). Groups that directly publish the data from the laboratory to the dashboard (e.g., WastewaterSCAN) show substantially less lag in data availability compared to aggregated networks that rely on other groups to upload data before it can be displayed (e.g., NWSS). The lag shown in Figure 4-15 was also affected by sampling interval, which was also shorter in WastewaterSCAN. However, across all networks, data timeliness was similar across levels of Social Vulnerability

---

[13] See https://www.cdc.gov/vaccines/programs/iis/about.html.

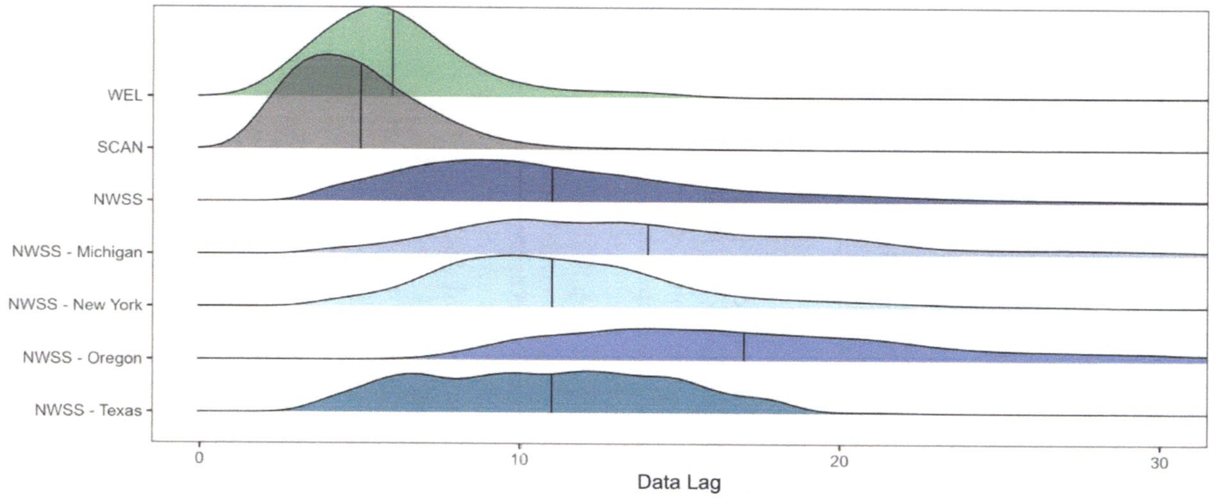

FIGURE 4-15 Evaluation of the timeliness of SARS-CoV-2 data over 2 months from (top to bottom) a local university laboratory dashboard (Wigginton-Eisenberg Lab [WEL]), WastewaterSCAN (SCAN), and NWSS, including several example states within NWSS (Michigan, New York, Oregon, and Texas). These example states span a range of population sizes, total area, and wastewater program scales, to illustrate the potential variation in data lag state by state. The data lag indicates how many days old the most recently available data are (i.e., the current date at the time the website was checked, minus the sampling date for the most recent posted data). Groups that directly publish the data from laboratory to dashboard (WEL and SCAN) show substantially less lag in data availability compared to aggregated networks that rely on other groups to upload data before it can be displayed (such as NWSS and various component states within NWSS). Line is the median.
SOURCE: J. Gilbert and M. Eisenberg, University of Michigan, personal communication, 2024.

Index and across urban-rural categories, suggesting that while data timeliness may be an issue for some sites, it does not appear correlated with communities' socioeconomic status or rurality (J. Gilbert and M. Eisenberg, University of Michigan, personal communication, 2024).

Given the data lags of more than 2 weeks in aggregate networks such as NWSS, new timing requirements for reporting would enhance actionability of wastewater surveillance. Additionally, improvements in data submission processes, including allowing for provisional data submission and increasing automation of data reporting, including wastewater treatment plant flow data, would reduce data lags and enhance the timeliness of public health response.

ADVANCING STATISTICAL TOOLS FOR INTERPRETATION AND PREDICTION

The expansion of wastewater surveillance during the pandemic brought with it advances in the use of models to understand wastewater data, building on earlier efforts more focused on enteric pathogens. Wastewater data are particularly of interest for modeling and forecasting efforts due to their potential for providing leading data, compared to hospitalizations or deaths. Recent research has worked to advance the capacity of models to use wastewater surveillance data to better estimate current underlying disease incidence or prevalence (i.e., nowcasting; Klaassen et al., 2024; Lai et al., 2023), and effective reproductive numbers (Nadeau et al., 2024) and to improve the accuracy of epidemiological forecasting tools (e.g., Polcz et al., 2023; Vaughan et al., 2023). Modeling tools are also beginning to be used to extrapolate wastewater data to understand disease trends in rural areas located outside of monitored sewersheds (Meadows et al., 2024). Finally, modeling can also play a role in evaluation and guidance of interventions and decision making informed by wastewater data; models can be used to assess "what if" scenarios, alternative response strategies, and counterfactuals, such as how the timing of detection or decision making might have unfolded differently with versus without wastewater monitoring.

Wastewater data have recently been incorporated into COVID-19 forecasting models produced by CDC[14] and the Public Health Agency of Canada (Joung et al., 2023). CDC has made sizable investments in this area through its Center for Forecasting and Outbreak Analytics[15] and recently granted $262 million in funding to develop disease forecasting methods and tools,

---

[14] See https://www.cdc.gov/forecast-outbreak-analytics/about/wastewater-informed-forecasting.html.

[15] See https://www.cdc.gov/forecast-outbreak-analytics/index.html.

test them at the pilot scale, and ultimately scale up to deploy these tools at larger scales (CDC, 2023c).

The types of models being used range from statistical models (e.g., linear regression [Leisman et al., 2024], score-based models [Usmani et al., 2024]), to more complex statistical and machine learning models (Lai et al., 2023; Vaughan et al., 2023), to mechanistic models (Phan et al., 2023). Mechanistic models explicitly model various processes such as transmission, infection, pathogen shedding, and transport in the sewer system, and their prediction accuracy depends upon accurate information on these various processes. In contrast, statistical and machine learning tools do not depend on an understanding of processes; instead, they discern trends and predict probable outcomes using large data sets. As such, future disease transmission is assumed to behave the same as in past data sets (i.e., stationarity). These differences often give mechanistic models some advantages when it comes to prediction in new circumstances (e.g., simulating what-if scenarios or possible intervention strategies) and allow the models to be more explainable and interpretable. However, machine learning models typically have more advantage for pure forecasting due to their greater flexibility and lower reliance on assumptions about structure. Machine learning tools can also draw upon diverse data sets that may provide less-obvious information to help inform aspects of the model related to the spread of disease (e.g., weather patterns).

Although there has been an explosion of wastewater modeling efforts in the past 4 years, the use of models to estimate prevalence or predict epidemiological metrics such as cases, hospitalizations, and deaths is still in its infancy. To improve the use of models to understand incidence and prevalence and strengthen forecasting capabilities, numerous data needs exist:

- Publicly available, raw (non-normalized) wastewater surveillance data for many sewersheds across different geographic areas, sewershed sizes, and other varying features, to provide large data sets for assessing modeling capabilities;
- Improvements in wastewater surveillance data quality and consistency (see also Chapters 2 and 3), to reduce nonintrinsic variability derived from differences sampling, processing, and analysis;
- Reduced lags in data reporting, which impact the predictive power of forecasting tools;
- Improved spatial data, including sewershed boundaries so that wastewater data can be accurately mapped to other geographic data sets by county or census tract;
- Shedding data for wastewater surveillance targets, including the distribution of shedding kinetics across a range of individuals and

the shape of that distribution for each target (and variant) by stage of the disease;
- Prospective epidemiological studies to validate mechanistic or statistical models (see Box 4-3); and
- Improved understanding of viral, bacterial, and fungal decay and loss of RNA and DNA signals in wastewater systems prior to sampling, including effect of travel times, temperature, and wastewater chemistry in a range of system sizes.

Additional developments in modeling and data integration tools could substantially advance efforts to triangulate and integrate wastewater data with other data sources. Models could provide a common mathematical and statistical framework for multiple distinct data types, enabling estimates and conclusions to be drawn from across these different sources—potentially mitigating some of the different biases present in each. As discussed earlier in this chapter, local health jurisdictions that have invested in data integration efforts to date rely mainly on plotting disparate data on the same plot or same page. Model-based analysis of disparate data sets would increase confidence in data interpretations and improve the reliability of disease forecasting, thereby improving local public health decisions while reducing staff burden. Advances in modeling tools that link machine learning with elements of mechanistic models (e.g., Chopra et al., 2023; Drake et al., 2023; Rodriguez et al., 2023) could draw upon the strengths of both approaches, bringing knowledge of component processes while also using machine learning to explore areas where such processes are poorly understood.

PUBLIC HEALTH RESPONSE GUIDANCE

As noted in the committee's previous report (NASEM, 2023) and according to the needs assessment conducted by the NWSS Centers of Excellence from Colorado and Houston (R. Schneider, Houston Health Department and K. Weisbeck, Colorado Department of Health, personal communication, 2024), local health departments continue to need support in understanding what actions they can take with wastewater surveillance data. Additional pathogen targets as well as different sampling approaches and population coverage (e.g., sampling at large citywide wastewater treatment plants, small plants, or facilities) make understanding how to respond to the data for public health intervention even more complicated. The response to detection of a target can differ based on a variety of factors including disease severity, stigma, and/or spreading rates. Depending upon these factors, targets may have different timelines for notifications of public health staff and different intervention approaches. The actions, as well

---

BOX 4-3
Moving from Trends to Estimating
Prevalence in the Community

While is it fairly well established that trends in respiratory viruses in wastewater correspond to the rise and fall of infections in the community, translation of these values to an empirical estimate of the number of people infected in the community remains a major challenge. Unlike hospitalizations or deaths that can provide known values to calibrate statistical models, the number of people infected at a point in time is difficult to determine. Mechanistic models could be used to estimate infection prevalence, but many knowledge gaps need to be filled. Among the multiple variables that could influence estimates in a mechanistic model, shedding rates are perhaps the most important to determine. For SARS-CoV-2, these can be highly variable depending on the individual (e.g., whether the individual is a super-shedder), stage of the disease, and likely by variants (Arts et al., 2023; F. Li et al., 2023; Prasek et al., 2023). Early studies showed that shedding rates of individuals could vary by up to four orders of magnitude (Zheng et al., 2020). Modeling of SARS-CoV-2 shedding in a community using clinical testing as the basis for estimating infection rates showed shedding can vary by almost two orders of magnitude and depending on age, demographics, or the variant circulation in the community (Prasek et al., 2022). Although some of the expansion targets under consideration (see Chapter 5) have shedding data, many do not, and what data sets exist may be incomplete for fully encompassing the variability of individuals across an outbreak. The large variation in shedding (e.g., super-shedder versus an asymptomatic/low shedder) is highly important to capture if transmission dynamics are to be accurately reflected in the models. Additionally, once the target enters the sewer system, temperature (Hart and Halden, 2020), transport times (Schussman and McLellan, 2022), partitioning to solids or settling (Ye et al., 2016), and other factors that affect decay of viruses and bacteria will influence the final concentrations of DNA or RNA recovered in a wastewater sample.

Prospective epidemiological studies could help validate mechanistic models or be used to develop statistical relationships between wastewater concentrations and the number of people infected. For example, ongoing respiratory surveillance cohorts (such as those already funded by CDC) could recruit participants in alignment with wastewater treatment plant catchment areas, enabling comparison between wastewater and epidemiological data on infection patterns (particularly for highly under-ascertained illnesses) and allowing for validation of mechanistic models. Such studies can also be used to evaluate shedding patterns (ideally by demographic variables such as age), which can be used to inform further modeling efforts. Prospective studies can also often capture asymptomatic, presymptomatic, and other less frequently detected infections (depending on their testing structure), making them particularly useful for validating wastewater monitoring, compared with clinical data that may only reflect symptomatic individuals.

as the response time, differ by location. For example, detection of RSV in wastewater from an assisted living facility with a population of elderly residents who are at risk for severe disease may trigger specific actions such as masking and spatial distancing within the facility while actions may differ for detection of the same target in a wastewater treatment plant covering a large population (e.g., messaging about the risk to infants as well as the elderly and emphasizing maternal as well as adult vaccination).

Development of national guidance for response actions by wastewater target and population coverage location would provide support for jurisdictions in their local decision making. Such a response framework reduces uncertainty about which actions are appropriate after the detection of a target, creating accountability and maximizing efficiency. For a given detected target, there will be a logical set of suggested responses that could be customized. This way each jurisdiction need not develop a plan independently. As an example, Komal et al. (2024) developed a framework for Houston that is adaptable for other jurisdictions according to their capacity. The plan addresses several additional wastewater targets for potential wastewater surveillance identified by a survey of local infectious disease doctors (Sheth et al., 2024a). It outlines clear internal health department notification timelines, who needs to be notified upon receiving a wastewater target detection or a spike above baseline, and what their action would be. The timelines, actions, and order of actions were derived through consultation with leaders of the various departments/programs in the public health agency. An example of application of this plan is outlined in Figure 4-16.

EVALUATING THE PUBLIC HEALTH VALUE OF THE WASTEWATER SURVEILLANCE SYSTEM

Expanding wastewater surveillance beyond the COVID-19 emergency involves costs, including monetary costs; workloads for utilities, local health jurisdictions, and CDC; and opportunity costs as leaders strive to meet those demands amidst resource scarcity. It also has the potential to yield significant public health benefits. Yet, that outcome is not guaranteed, and the currently available evidence does not permit quantification of the value of wastewater information relative to the investments required to generate it. Given the costs and resource scarcity within CDC, a plan for monitoring and evaluating the public health benefit of NWSS should be set in place once the key decisions about the system's design over the next 5–8 years are made.

This evaluation plan should cover several dimensions of program success. First, technical success: are the chosen sampling design, targets, and analytical methods yielding the expected information (or better) at the expected level of confidence (or better)? Second, usefulness: do stakeholders

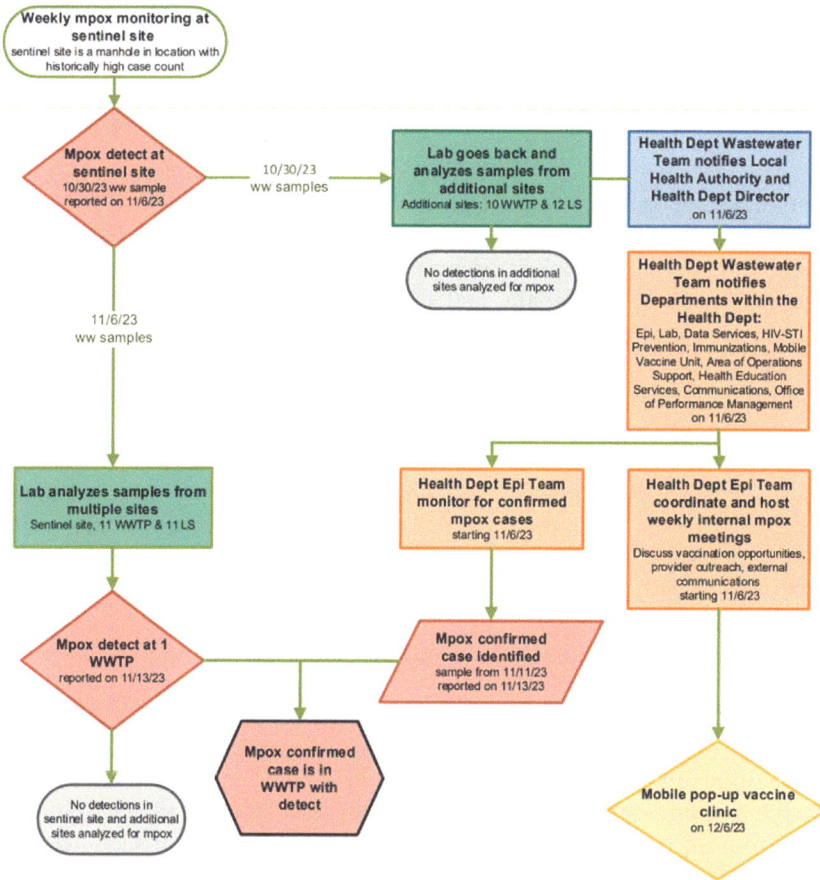

FIGURE 4-16 A decision-making framework for the City of Houston for Mpox, with dates from a recent detection and related response actions included. Similar frameworks could be provided as models for NWSS targets to provide guidance for state, local, and tribal public health jurisdictions.
SOURCE: Adapted from Sheth et al., 2024b.

perceive the wastewater data to substantially improve their ability to make public health decisions? This involves assessing both the marginal utility of wastewater data relative to other available sources of surveillance data and people's ability to actually act on the data in ways that prevent morbidity and mortality. Third, what burdens does participating in NWSS involve? Burdens may be material (e.g., resources, staff time) or more intangible (e.g., stigmatization, fatigue). Fourth, in system participants' view, does the value of the information outweigh the burdens? That assessment requires looking back at the public health wins the system has supported, as well as forward to the harms it seems likely to make meaningful contributions to averting in the future.

DATA ACCESS FOR RESEARCH

Expanding access to community-level NWSS data has substantial potential benefits for facilitating research and informing public health action. Throughout a range of contexts in public health, calls have emerged for more open data, metadata, and statistical code, recognizing the potential scientific gains associated with broadly sharing these building blocks of research innovation (IOM, 2015; Ross et al., 2023). Data sharing (with appropriate measures to protect data security and individual privacy) has become an accepted and expected part of research in many health fields, from clinical trials to genomics to health economics, even though the data sets may involve sensitive, individual-level data. Broad data access ensures "not simply that a single database can be used more widely, [but also] that these data can be leveraged, shared and combined with other datasets" (Huston et al., 2019). In other areas, such as immunization data, CDC has already taken steps to facilitate greater sharing of data across local health jurisdictions.[16] Among the motivations for these efforts is CDC's recognition that expanded access to data promotes health equity.[17]

Currently, health departments that submit data to NWSS cannot directly download data from sampling locations in other jurisdictions and cannot in any other way receive data that include specific geographic identifiers. CDC may facilitate communications among jurisdictions that would like to collaborate and share data but does not itself supply other jurisdictions' data. Other interested persons, including academic researchers and private companies working in the predictive analytics space, may submit a request to CDC to receive data and metadata (i.e., the full 200 analytic variables in the NWSS database) from community-level sampling sites, after executing a data use agreement. The data include state and county information but not the exact address or name of the sampling location. Tribal data and data from sites with a population under 3,000 are not shared (K. Cesa, CDC, personal communication, 2024).

CDC's data sharing policies represent an effort to balance data access with the need to protect and nurture CDC's relationship with the health departments contributing data. Health departments may be concerned that sharing data openly with precise geographic identifiers could lead to

---

[16] See https://www.cdc.gov/surveillance/data-modernization/snapshot/2022-snapshot/stories/transforming-immunization-data.html.

[17] See https://www.cdc.gov/surveillance/data-modernization/dmi-health-equity.html.

stigmatization of communities where pathogen levels are relatively high or loss of public trust in the health department or local and national wastewater surveillance systems. Although the committee is not aware of evidence that any stigmatization has arisen from community-level wastewater surveillance, maintaining community trust and participation requires solicitude to the risk. Facility- or institution-level wastewater data (as opposed to community-level data) may involve a nontrivial risk of identifying individuals or creating stigma (see also NASEM, 2023).

Another argument in favor of stringent controls on data access is that most data uses that fit the definition of public health *surveillance*, as opposed to research, will not undergo ethical review by an institutional review board (Otto et al., 2014). Data sharing in other areas, such as clinical trials, has also raised concerns that, even if metadata are provided, secondary users may not understand how to use data in a way that generates scientifically valid results. This is a particular concern where secondary users seek to combine data from multiple primary sources in a single analysis and may not appreciate differences across data sets that make them noncomparable—a circumstance that arises for wastewater data. Finally, some data contributors to the NWSS may have executed data use agreements that did not contemplate broad data sharing and would require updating.

Yet, restrictive data sharing policies come at a cost. Specific geographic identifiers are crucial to conducting wastewater-based epidemiological analysis and creating forecasting models. The ability to use detailed geographic information and metadata may facilitate the discovery of underlying features of particular infectious diseases that could reduce future health impacts. For example, is there a trend to higher population occurrence (as implied by wastewater measurements) for individuals in certain air pollution nonattainment areas, when corrected for potential confounding variables? Geographic data help analysts understand who is and is not represented in the NWSS, how pathogen levels vary across sites, how trends in pathogen levels converge or diverge across geographic areas over time, and how well a forecasting model fits actual wastewater data from different geographic areas. Making data easy to access facilitates inclusion of more researchers in efforts to formulate and test different strategies and concepts—efforts that may not be undertaken if they involve an arduous process of applying for permission to use data or if the necessary data are wholly unavailable. An additional benefit of facilitating wide access to data is that researchers not otherwise included within the traditional framework of users (e.g., molecular biologists, engineers, sociologists, geographers) may have knowledge of or access to other data sets and sources of information that can be fused with the wastewater data to generate novel insights that could advance the field.

To balance communities' concerns with the benefits of broader data access, the committee recommends that CDC provide community-level wastewater data with site identifiers to researchers or other public health jurisdictions through an expeditious process while maintaining some degree of control over how NWSS data are used. This recommendation would appear to be aligned with the broad goals of CDC's recently updated Public Health Data Strategy,[18] but it is unclear what specific plans CDC envisions for wastewater data. The committee suggests a data sharing process with four hallmarks:

1. Requests for data use should be individually assessed. The committee's Phase 1 report (NASEM, 2023) described how an ethics advisory committee could be constituted by CDC and tasked with reviewing applications for data uses. This ethics advisory committee, which could be modeled after existing committees reviewing secondary data uses at universities, would be given the remit of determining whether data use requests hold promise for generating a scientific and/or public health benefit and whether risks (including the risk of community stigmatization given public concern about the pathogen) are minimized through data handling procedures and reasonable in relation to the anticipated benefits. In addition to recommending approval or disapproval of requests, the ethics advisory committee would be empowered to work with requestors to strengthen data use proposals by describing specific measures to ensure adequate protection of the data and of the communities that have contributed the data. The ethics advisory committee should be transparent with NWSS data depositors and the public about the criteria used to assess requests.

2. Data requestors should be required to execute a data use agreement. Where public health data have identifying information attached and are considered to be even somewhat sensitive, it is appropriate to commit those who access them to basic terms of responsible use. This includes consulting metadata (e.g., detection limits, sampling method and frequency, treatment plan population coverage, laboratory analytical methods) to understand aspects of the data that may make particular analyses or statistical approaches not scientifically valid. Doing so promotes public trust and ensures that the "ground rules" of the data sharing are respected.

3. The data use agreement should be short, simple, unified, and standardized. Data requestors should sign one data use agreement with CDC, rather than individual agreements with contributing sites.

---

[18] See https://www.cdc.gov/ophdst/public-health-data-strategy/index.html.

Further, the data use agreement template should reflect the principle that the amount of legal architecture around a data transfer should be commensurate with the level of risk and sensitivity of the data. Community-level wastewater data—even with site identifiers—are fairly low-risk data, both in terms of the sensitivity of information they convey about individuals and small areas and in terms of the potential consequences for individuals and communities were the confidentiality of the data breached. Data use agreements should bind data users to (1) not share data with third parties; (2) not publish results that identify specific wastewater treatment plant data by name or make specific treatment plants readily identifiable; and (3) use data only to conduct the analyses specified in the data use application, returning to CDC for further permission if they would like to explore additional analyses. Bearing in mind that executing data use agreements within universities is often a protracted process and that delays tend to arise from haggling over other kinds of provisions, such as indemnification (Mello et al., 2020), limiting wastewater data use agreements to these three basic terms will help ensure that the process facilitates rather than impedes research.

4. Periodic reassessment of the data access policy should be part of the work of CDC's data ethics committee (Mello et al., 2023; NASEM, 2023). Most importantly, a decision to shift the scale of wastewater data collection or analysis from the community level to more targeted surveillance should trigger reconsideration of current policy. The committee's Phase 1 report (NASEM, 2023) described several other conditions that also should prompt a fresh look at whether the current policy still represents the optimal balance between data access and protection of other interests. These include advances in reidentification techniques, a court ruling that wastewater data are more discoverable or admissible in legal proceedings than previously understood, changes in the degree of stigmatization or other risks associated with finding a high level of a pathogen in a specific community, and any reports of unexpected data uses, such as access by law enforcement.

CDC should make NWSS contributors aware of the shift in policy, describe participation in the data sharing program as a condition of NWSS participation, update agreements with contributors as needed, and describe how CDC safeguards data confidentiality and protects against misuse. It should also explain the benefits of sharing geographic identifiers—both for contributing health departments, which may now conduct comparisons with other jurisdictions much more easily, and for wastewater science generally. When external researchers achieve important advances (e.g., in modeling) based on NWSS data, these innovations should be communicated to local health departments to demonstrate the ongoing value of contributing and sharing data. Over the longer term, continued conversation with NWSS participants that have expressed reservations about greater data sharing may help CDC move toward providing public access to community-level wastewater data without the need for data use agreements.

Local health departments, in turn, should send regular communications to their wastewater treatment plant partners, sharing back wastewater surveillance results and broader advances in the field of wastewater surveillance that have been made possible through WWTPs' contributions. Helping WWTP staff understand the value of wastewater surveillance to public health action can ensure strong, continued partnerships as the exigencies of the COVID-19 pandemic fade.

CONCLUSIONS AND RECOMMENDATIONS

Further analysis is urgently needed to resolve uncertainty about whether normalization improves data quality and comparability and, if so, to identify a cohesive approach to normalization in the NWSS. Ideally, data normalization would aid comparison of data across sites and reduce variability at a single site, but normalization also has the potential to introduce significant additional variability into the reported results. Currently, there is no scientific consensus regarding which normalization factors or approaches perform best under various conditions, and no single normalization approach has been identified that improves data quality and comparability in wastewater surveillance data at a national scale. The NWSS currently presents data with inconsistent normalization approaches, which complicates interpretations across sites. NWSS leadership should develop a clear rationale for data normalization and a robust process to evaluate multiple factors. Research using large, existing data sets and data science techniques is needed to determine whether to normalize and, if so, using which method(s).

The NWSS should advance plug-and-play tools and, in the near term, provide open-source code for advanced analytical tools that provide public health agencies with nationally consistent data analysis and visualization approaches that contextualize risk. The NWSS has made substantial advancements in its public-facing dashboard, but many states and localities still prefer using their local dashboards with their own customized data analytics. Yet, the variability in data analysis approaches across states makes it difficult for localities to readily compare their observations to others. Although some states may initially prefer to continue using their own individually developed analytic approaches, as new pathogen targets are added, the burden of data analysis, visualization, and interpretation will only continue to increase. The long-term goal is for the NWSS to provide plug-and-play tools and overarching metrics that are easy to use and understand and substantially reduce the burden on localities to develop, interpret, and contextualize their wastewater surveillance data. In the near term, CDC should work with partners to develop open-source code in a common programming language to help localities conduct advanced analytics using data downloaded from DCIPHER. To assist this effort, CDC could draw upon data analytics expertise and resources in its Centers of Excellence, large public health jurisdictions, and other federal agencies, such as the Environmental Protection Agency, U.S. Geological Survey, or the Centers for Medicare & Medicaid Services. Sharing the code with public health agencies will promote further improvement by end users.

Automated data entry and reporting deadlines would improve the timeliness of NWSS data. Currently, there are a range of workflow approaches, with substantial lag times between sample collection and data availability for some sites. Delays in sample processing and data entry impact the potential response of public health agencies to new outbreaks or disease spread. The NWSS should develop user-friendly data entry tools with automated quality checks for laboratories and wastewater treatment plants and require their use to reduce reporting delays. Laboratories should submit data within 48–72 hours after samples are received.

Improved data integration would significantly enhance the value of NWSS data. CDC should strive to integrate and improve sources of clinical data in its wastewater visualization tools and disease forecasting models so that public health agencies can better understand the larger context for the wastewater data, strengthen forecast predictions, and increase confidence in their public health actions. Databases already exist with information on immunization rates, emergency department syndromic surveillance, and reportable diseases, but these databases are not integrated with one another nor with wastewater surveillance and the data can be disparate or incomplete. Recent developments in modeling, machine learning, and data science offer important opportunities to integrate and gain insights across the data streams (including clinical testing, hospitalizations, and deaths).

To strengthen infectious disease forecasting and nowcasting using wastewater surveillance data, key information needs should be addressed. Priority information needs include

- Access to non-normalized data from NWSS sampling sites,
- Data on shedding rates (and their distribution) for NWSS targets,
- Improved geospatial data for monitored sewersheds,
- Improved understanding of pathogen decay in sewersheds, and
- Prospective epidemiological studies to validate mechanistic or statistical models.

These data would also help to extrapolate NWSS data to communities that are currently unrepresented in the NWSS. Pathogen shedding and decay data and prospective epidemiological studies will require major research investments to advance this foundational information upon which data interpretations can improve and expand. Pathogen evolution may affect shedding rates so these studies would need to be updated periodically. To be fully usefully applied, CDC will also need to reduce sources of variability from sampling, processing, and analysis, as described in Chapters 2 and 3.

CDC should adopt an expeditious process for making community-level wastewater data with site identifiers and associated metadata directly available to health departments and researchers upon request. The potential scientific benefits of broadening data sharing exceed the risks. However, given that some communities that contribute to the NWSS may be concerned about stigmatization and other risks, an unrestricted data access policy is not optimal for maintaining trust. Rather, CDC should convene an ethics advisory committee to review applications for data use by assessing the risk/benefit balance of the proposed use and the adequacy of the proposed data security and confidentiality procedures. Those granted access should execute a simple, standardized data use agreement with CDC containing three provisions: users will use data only to conduct the analyses specified in the data use application, will not share data with third parties, and will not publish results identifying specific wastewater treatment plants by name or making them readily identifiable. CDC should periodically reassess this data sharing policy in light of any new developments that bear on the risk/benefit balance of sharing. Due to identifiability concerns, facility-level data should not be included in the data sharing scheme. Over time, CDC should work with communities that have expressed concerns about publicly sharing their wastewater data to address those concerns so that data access can be further expanded, since even simplified data use agreements constitute a barrier to researchers entering the field.

CDC should develop guidance and model response action plans to help state, local, and tribal public health agencies understand the significance of changing infectious disease metrics and examples of actions that may be appropriate to further reduce risks. Although NASEM (2023) noted many examples of public health actions supported by wastewater surveillance data—often supported by related data sources—other small public health agencies that operate with limited staff have noted that the data are underused or only presented to the public without use in public health decision making. These agencies need assistance in understanding the significance of data presented by the NWSS to increase their capacity to reduce public health risks. This guidance is likely to differ for the various classes of organisms and evolve as the data integration and model forecasting capabilities improve.

CDC should develop a monitoring and evaluation plan for the NWSS that would be implemented once the key decisions about its design over the next 5–8 years are finalized. The plan should specify the information that needs to be collected to assess the key dimensions of *technical success*, *usefulness*, *burdens*, and whether the *value of the information* outweighs the burdens. The technical success assessment should include consideration of whether newly available technologies or methods could further enhance performance. The usefulness and value-of-information assessments should consider both the ways wastewater data have contributed to past public health actions and the potential for future benefit. The usefulness assessment should also consider whether the chosen list of targets has proved to be over- or underinclusive. The burden assessment should consider both tangible and intangible burdens. As with other research, collaboration with academic researchers is likely to be helpful in designing and implementing the evaluation plan.

5

Potential Target Expansion for National Endemic Disease Surveillance

In this chapter, the committee discusses the potential expansion of endemic targets for national wastewater surveillance. Over the past 12–18 months, the Centers for Disease Control and Prevention (CDC) has been actively exploring options for expanding endemic targets in the National Wastewater Surveillance System (NWSS) beyond COVID-19. The NWSS added Mpox monitoring (see Figure 4-7) and is piloting analysis of two other respiratory viruses targets—respiratory syncytial virus (RSV) and influenza A/B. If added to the NWSS core panel, all sites that use the national laboratory contract for analysis (i.e., approximately 9 percent of NWSS sites) would have their samples analyzed for these pathogens. Sites that conduct their own laboratory analyses could choose whether to analyze for the new pathogen targets. WastewaterSCAN,[1] which represents approximately 12 percent of NWSS sites, is currently analyzing 10 pathogen targets in addition to SARS-CoV-2: influenza, RSV, human metapneumovirus, parainfluenza, norovirus GIII, rotavirus, enterovirus D68, Mpox, *Candida auris*, and hepatitis A. The data from WastewaterSCAN surveillance will be extremely helpful in decision making and prioritizing additional targets for the NWSS in terms of analytical feasibility, correlation with population disease incidence, and public health action. This chapter discusses the potential value of specific targets under consideration for inclusion in the NWSS at a national scale as well as research needs for broad implementation.

In general, the additional endemic pathogens under consideration within the NWSS for national-scale surveillance include common respiratory

---

[1] See https://www.wastewaterscan.org/en/pathogens.

pathogens, enteric pathogens, and antimicrobial resistance genes. While respiratory and enteric infections may be seasonal or confined to localized outbreaks, their prevalence is sufficiently common in the United States to be considered endemic. Emerging pathogens with epidemic or pandemic potential (e.g., H5N1 avian influenza) and those causing sporadic, localized, or regional outbreaks (e.g., dengue virus, Mpox) are addressed in Chapter 6.

The committee's first report (NASEM, 2023) identified three criteria by which new targets should be evaluated: (1) the public health significance of the target, (2) analytical feasibility, including whether pathogen detection can be calibrated to public health outcomes of interest, and (3) the usefulness of community-level surveillance data to inform public health action (see Figure 5-1). Although existing wastewater surveillance samples could be analyzed for additional targets, the committee recognizes that the decision to implement additional targets will depend on available resources for laboratory analysis, data analysis, data visualization, and public health interpretation. It was beyond the task for the committee to conduct a formal evaluation of the value relative to the costs.

CURRENT AND POTENTIAL
RESPIRATORY VIRUS TARGETS

As of early 2024, two respiratory viruses (RSV and influenza A and B [flu]) were under active consideration by the U.S. Centers for Disease Control and Prevention (CDC) for incorporation in the NWSS in addition to SARS-CoV-2. At the same time, WastewaterSCAN was monitoring for six classes of respiratory viruses nationally: SARS-CoV-2, RSV, influenza A and B, human metapneumovirus, and parainfluenza, and enterovirus D68 (EVD68). SARS-CoV-2, RSV, and influenza A and B (flu) are logical targets for ongoing wastewater-based infectious disease surveillance because they satisfy all three criteria in the committee's first report for prioritizing pathogen targets (Figure 5-1), including that wastewater surveillance data add value for public health action relative to other existing methods of public health surveillance.

Now that routine clinical surveillance of SARS-CoV-2 has ceased, continued wastewater surveillance provides the primary ongoing epidemiological insight, beyond later-stage metrics such as hospitalizations and deaths, for a disease that continues to cause a significant public health burden. The evolution of the SARS-CoV-2 virus, however, may alter the infection and shedding dynamics within the population and necessitates ongoing recalibration of viral loads in wastewater to hospitalization or mortality data to ensure proper interpretation and public health action.

RSV and flu are major contributors to the annual respiratory disease burden and have had analytical feasibility demonstrated in several

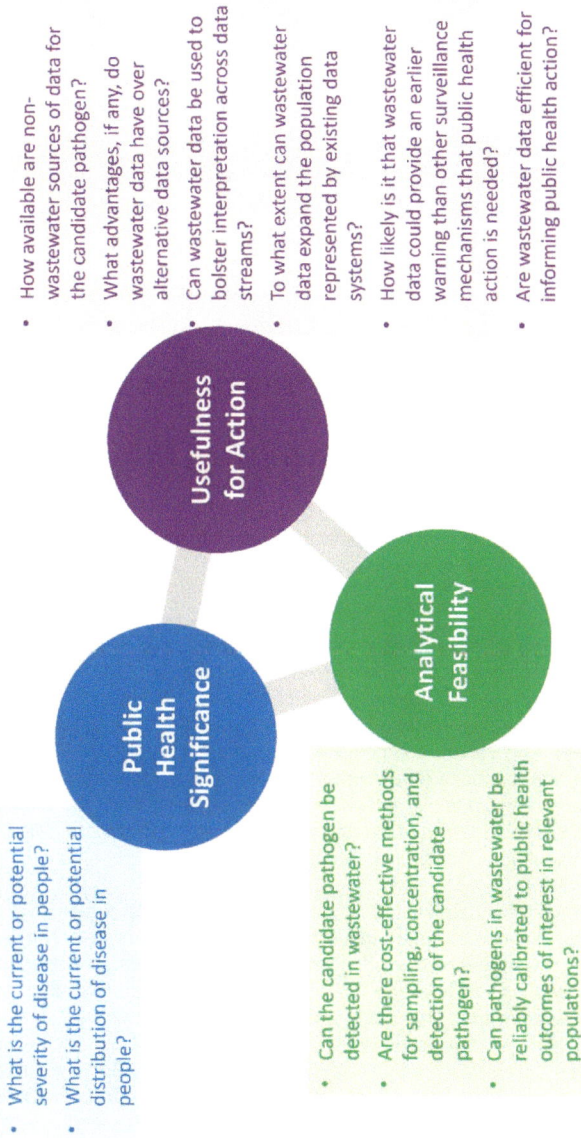

FIGURE 5-1 Framework for identifying candidate pathogens for wastewater surveillance.
SOURCE: NASEM, 2023.

wastewater settings (see Box 5-1). Given the seasonality of RSV and flu, wastewater surveillance can provide local data on increasing levels early in the annual cycle. Although RSV and flu are screened with respiratory panels in the clinical setting, these tests are not consistently ordered. Further, data that are collected vary by state and are not compiled for routine ongoing disease surveillance on a broad scale in the United States.

As discussed in Box 5-1, EVD68—a normally mild respiratory illness with the potential to cause a rare but severe neurological disorder leading to muscle weakness or paralysis in children—may also have promise for wastewater surveillance. However, additional information is needed to determine the value of the data for public health action.

BOX 5-1
Current and Potential Respiratory Virus Targets

The following summarizes what is known for several respiratory viruses with respect to the committee's three criteria for expanding National Wastewater Surveillance System (NWSS) targets shown in Figure 5-1. As of June 2024, NWSS was monitoring for SARS-CoV-2, with pilot testing for Respiratory Syncytial Viruses (RSV) and influenza A and B, and WastewaterSCAN was monitoring for SARS-CoV-2, RSV, influenza A and B, and enterovirus D68 (EVD68).

SARS-CoV-2 variants. Since the emergence and spread of SARS-CoV-2 in late 2019, new variants have continuously emerged—a pattern that is predicted to continue in the foreseeable future. As diagnostic testing and results reporting of non-hospitalized individuals has decreased over time, wastewater surveillance of both trends in SARS-CoV-2 viral levels and variant composition continues to be relevant for public health communication and response (NASAEM, 2023). *The detection of increasing levels of emergent variants in wastewater provides data for updating vaccines to include predominant variants and, when linked to emergency department and hospitalization data, improves understanding of variant virulence.*

Influenza viruses. Influenza A and B viruses are responsible for a high level of annual severe respiratory disease. The two influenza virus types differ in their temporal spread and peak infection levels as well as affecting different age groups. Vaccination protects against influenza A and B; however the efficacy of vaccination in protecting against infection and disease varies depending on the seasonally prevalent strain, especially for influenza A. Influenza A cases caused by specific strains of concern as well as mortality data are collected as a nationally notifiable condition.[a] Both influenza A and B are detectable in municipal wastewater settings, including the ability to assess trends in viral loads (DeJonge et al., 2023; Hughes et al., 2022; Mercier et al., 2022; Wolfe et al., 2022). Although influenza viruses can be screened with respiratory panels in the clinical setting, these tests are not consistently ordered and may lag behind detection

POTENTIAL ENTERIC PATHOGEN TARGETS

The four enteric pathogens that have been discussed publicly by CDC for potential inclusion in the NWSS at a national scale are adenovirus types F40 and 41, Shiga-toxin-producing *E. coli* (STEC), *Campylobacter*, and norovirus. WastewaterSCAN is currently surveilling adenovirus group F (including both F40 and F41 types), norovirus, and rotavirus. Detection of these three viral targets were associated with clinical positivity data (Ammerman et al., 2024; Boehm et al., 2024; Kazmer et al., 2024). Both the viral targets (adenovirus group F, norovirus, rotavirus) and the bacterial targets (STEC and *Campylobacter*) generally meet the first two National

---

in wastewater. Notably, wastewater levels of influenza A specifically have been shown to positively associate with clinical testing data (Boehm et al., 2023a).

RSV. Similar to flu and coronaviruses, RSV causes respiratory symptoms that range from mild to severe; infants, the elderly, and those with compromised immunity or pulmonary function are at the greatest risk for severe disease. RSV has two primary subtypes, A and B, which can circulate separately or concomitantly. Unlike influenza and SARS-CoV-1, RSV strains appear to be genetically stable, and the approved vaccines protect against both RSV A and B. Analytics can detect both types and can distinguish between RSV A and B. Similar to wastewater detection of influenza and SARS-CoV-2, RSV levels in wastewater positively associate with clinical laboratory data (Boehm et al., 2023a; Zulli et al., 2024). Temporally, wastewater detection of RSV appears to most commonly peak concomitantly with clinical peaks, although wastewater detection has preceded clinical detection in a subset of municipalities surveyed (Zulli et al., 2024). Notably, wastewater surveillance can distinguish between RSV A and B, which is not typically done at the clinical level, and provide data related to transmissibility and virulence of the predominant subtype (Zambrana et al., 2024).

Enterovirus D68 (EVD68). EVD68 has been responsible for regular outbreaks of a polio-like illness (acute flaccid myelitis) in children since 2014. Several groups have already demonstrated the analytical feasibility of wastewater surveillance for EVD68 (Boehm et al., 2023b; Pelligrinelli et al., 2023; Tedcastle et al., 2022; Weil et al., 2017), and the wastewater trend data have been shown to correlate with clinical diagnoses (Erster et al., 2022). Retrospective analyses of wastewater samples from Colorado indicated enterovirus D68 (EV-D68) was detected well-ahead of syndromic or clinical laboratory signals. As a result, Colorado public health officials implemented wastewater testing for EV-D68 as part of its enterovirus surveillance model as an early warning system for healthcare surge planning during respiratory virus season. The inclusion of EVD68 in the WastewaterSCAN surveillance can provide data as to the value of incorporation into the NWSS to public health action.

---

[a] See https://www.cdc.gov/flu/weekly/overview.htm.

Academies' (NASEM, 2023) prioritization criteria—public health signifi-cance and analytical feasibility (see Figure 5-1 and Box 5-2). All cause significant health effects, and most have little other consistent clinical sur-veillance data. As enteric pathogens, each of these is shed readily into wastewater at relatively high levels (Kosulin et al., 2016; Lenaker et al., 2024; Teunis et al., 2014), and analytical quantification of adenoviruses, noroviruses, rotavirus, and *Campylobacter* in wastewater has been shown to be feasible. Additional research on the specificity of polymerase chain reaction (PCR)-based detection of STEC may be needed because the tar-geted Shiga-toxin genes may not always indicate presence in pathogenic *E. coli*. Shiga-toxin genes may be detected that are not expressed or are not

---

BOX 5-2
Current and Potential Enteric Pathogen Targets

The following summarizes what is known for several enteric pathogen targets with respect to the committee's three criteria for expanding NWSS targets shown in Figure 5-1. Of these, as of June 2024, WastewaterSCAN was monitoring for Adenovirus types F40 and 41 and norovirus.

Adenovirus. Numerous strains of adenovirus exist, with most being respiratory patho-gens. Types F40 and 41 differ in that they have primarily been associated as a sig-nificant cause of diarrheal disease (Ghebremedhin, 2014). These strains were also associated with an unusual outbreak of pediatric hepatitis in 2022, raising concerns of their public health significance (Wollants et al., 2022). No routine passive surveil-lance or active clinical surveillance exists for adenovirus types F40 and 41, although studies have described its detection in wastewater demonstrating analytical feasibility (Allayeh et al., 2022; Boehm et al., 2024; Jothikumar et al., 2005; Pérez-Zabaleta et al., 2022). The potential for wastewater surveillance data to inform public health action is currently unknown.

Norovirus. Norovirus is a very common cause of diarrhea, with endemic and epidemic strains, that is not included as an individual notifiable condition for CDC. It is commonly implicated in food and waterborne outbreaks and is, therefore, passively captured as an implicated etiologic agent in notifiable food and water outbreaks.[a] Individual cases are generally not reported, but several states participate in voluntary surveillance for outbreaks.[b] Numerous studies have quantified norovirus in wastewater and correlated it with other epidemiological surveillance data, thus demonstrating the value in using wastewater to track community infection trends (Ammerman et al., 2024; Boehm et al., 2023c). With a short incubation period and disease typically self-resolving in 24–72 hours, implementation of public health interventions for norovirus outside of an out-break setting may prove difficult, although wastewater could be used to inform changes in cleaning practices in facilities that may be more likely to experience outbreaks (e.g., residence halls, childcare settings).

functional (cryptic copies) or are carried in bacteriophage rather than *E. coli*, and therefore would require confirmation by selective culture.

Prior to national implementation, additional testing would be informative to demonstrate the extent to which these data can inform meaningful health actions or interventions, given the timing of each illness and the nature of disease spread relative to the timing of wastewater surveillance. The committee supports the rollout of these agents at a limited number of NWSS sites or analysis of public health response from the WastewaterSCAN data, supported by the NWSS Centers of Excellence, to further explore the value of national data collection on enteric pathogens for public health action. A limited rollout could assess whether wastewater surveillance of

Shiga-toxin-producing *E. coli* (STEC). STEC is a common foodborne bacterial pathogen that results in a bloody diarrhea and is occasionally implicated in waterborne outbreaks. STEC is associated with serious sequelae (e.g., Guillain-Barré syndrome, hemolytic uremic syndrome; Blaser, 2004), and CDC lists STEC as a notifiable condition.[a] Considering the temporal elements of disease and the exposure pathways most commonly associated with STEC transmission, the temporality of wastewater data may not add benefit over passive case surveillance.

Campylobacter. *Campylobacter* is also a common foodborne bacterial pathogen and is a very prevalent etiologic agent of bacterial diarrheal disease. Like STEC, *Campylobacter* is associated with serious sequelae and is a notifiable condition.[a] A recent meta-analysis suggests wastewater surveillance of *Campylobacter* is analytically feasible (Zhang et al., 2023a), although degradation of the *Campylobacter* signal in wastewater may confound association with caseload (Zhang et al., 2023b). The capacity for wastewater surveillance data to inform public health action is currently unknown.

Salmonella. *Salmonella* is responsible for more hospitalizations than all other foodborne diseases (Dewey-Mattia et al., 2018). Research has shown that clinical cases of salmonellosis were correlated with *Salmonella* in wastewater (Yan et al., 2018), but there are a large number of *Salmonella* strains from different sources that are shed in wastewater, complicating interpretation of detection at the genus level. Analytical methods that would allow strain-level delineation of *Salmonella* levels in wastewater may be technically challenging, although culture-based methods could fulfill this need. Detection of disease-causing strains of *Salmonella* in wastewater could support public communication and actions to prevent future exposures.

---

[a] See https://www.cdc.gov/nndss/index.html.
[b] See https://www.cdc.gov/norovirus/reporting/index.html.

these targets can provide sufficiently timely information such that actions could be implemented to alter community-level pathogen dynamics (e.g., advising increased handwashing and increased cleaning at schools). These pilots could also inform the development of guidance for local public health jurisdictions on how to interpret these new data (see also Chapter 4). Even if the surveillance data prove to be not timely enough to mitigate localized outbreaks, the pilot could determine whether the data can be useful to understand the community-scale disease trends over time to inform future public health actions or increase knowledge of disease dynamics in the community to a degree that justifies the investment. This approach with support from academic partners can minimize unnecessary burden on public health agency staff to interpret the data until the value for public health action is determined and guidance and messaging plans are available.

An additional enteric target candidate with potential is *Salmonella*, which has great public health significance. It is a highly prevalent foodborne pathogen, second to norovirus as the most confirmed etiology for foodborne infections in the United States (and above both STEC and *Campylobacter*). If technical challenges could be resolved allowing detection of disease-causing strains (see Box 5-2), wastewater surveillance of *Salmonella* may allow local health care jurisdictions to better communicate foodborne disease risks in their communities.

ANTIBIOTIC RESISTANCE GENE TARGETS

Four classes of antimicrobial resistance genes have been considered for potential inclusion in the NWSS: carbapenamases, extended spectrum β-lactamases (ESBLs), colistin resistance, and vancomycin resistance (see Box 5-3). Each of these targets has public health significance and maps to the National Action Plan for Combatting Antibiotic Resistant Bacteria 2020–2025 (Federal Task Force for Combating Antibiotic-Resistant Bacteria, 2020).

Although these antibiotic resistance genes can be detected in municipal wastewater, the interpretation of the data with respect to public health is by no means straightforward. Antibiotic resistance can be naturally occurring (intrinsic) in certain bacterial strains (notably with colistin resistance), acquired by chromosomal changes in genes (e.g., mutations), or acquired through mobile genetic elements. In fact, antibiotic resistance genes are frequently found on plasmids or other mobile elements that enhance their spread and can be detected in organisms in community wastewater (Hackenberger et al., 2024). Because there is no single antibiotic resistance gene target for major classes of resistance, detection of the full range of antibiotic resistance genes will require using multiple assays.

BOX 5-3
Potential Antibiotic Resistance Gene Targets

In public discussions, CDC has mentioned the following antibiotic resistance gene targets as possible future targets for future community wastewater surveillance, although no decisions have been made as of May 2024.

Carbapenemases and other extended spectrum β-lactamases (ESBLs) confer enzyme-mediated resistance to commonly used β-lactam antibiotics—such as carbapenem, penicillin, and cephalosporin—in a wide range of pathogens (e.g., *Klebsiella pneumoniae, Acinetobacter baumanii, Escherichia coli*) that cause common and severe hospital-acquired infections. Many of the ESBL gene targets are already widespread in the community; however, select genes targets for carbapenemase resistance are rarer and just beginning to emerge in the general population. An added complication is that several of the organisms in which these genes occur are opportunistic pathogens (e.g., environmental organisms that can infect compromised humans) and have been detected in wastewater systems.

Colistin resistance, particularly in multidrug-resistant Gram-negative bacteria within Enterobacterales and Pseudomonadales, is a major concern because colistin has been considered a last-line antibiotic treatment. Similar to the ESBLs, the genes that confer colistin resistance are in organisms that can be commonly found free-living in wastewater systems independent of human inputs.

Vancomycin resistance is a concern in Gram-positive pathogens such as *Staphylococcus,* enterococci, and *Clostridioides difficile* and is associated with severe hospital-acquired infections. As a result, the use of vancomycin has generally been limited to complicated infections due to concerns on the development or acquisition of resistance.

The presence of antibiotic resistance genes from nonhuman sources, the growth of antibiotic-resistant bacteria in biofilms within the sewage system, and the transfer of mobile genes within the environment may further confound any interpretation of wastewater antibiotic resistance gene prevalence at the community scale for public health and health system action. Consolidated wastewater streams may serve not just as a reservoir but also as an amplifier of antimicrobial resistance genes, making it difficult to relate the levels observed to carriage in the population. Culture approaches have shown *Aeromonas*, an abundant member of the microbial community of sewage (McLellan and Roguet, 2019), has a wide range of β-lactamase genes (Piotrawska et al., 2017), highlighting the importance of considering the contribution of resident microorganisms in wastewater systems to antibiotic resistance signals. Similarly, *Enterococcus* containing VanA, which confers vancomycin resistance, is also widespread in untreated wastewater (Liu et al., 2023). The committee expects wastewater surveillance to detect the already prevalent antibiotic resistance genes in nearly all community-level (i.e., wastewater treatment plant) samples. Therefore, at the community scale, wastewater surveillance data on antibiotic resistance gene occurrence cannot be reliably calibrated relative to public health outcomes of interest, and widespread monitoring at current NWSS wastewater treatment plant sampling sites is unlikely to be useful to inform public health actions.

In light of these confounding factors, as discussed in Chapter 2, facility-level antibiotic resistance gene monitoring would be more actionable than wastewater treatment plant monitoring. Facility wastewater is less likely to be confounded by nonhuman or environmental reservoirs of resistance genes, although this has yet to be tested. The detection or changes in levels of rare antibiotic resistance targets (e.g., rarer carbapenem and colistin resistance targets) in hospitals, skilled nursing facilities, and assisted living facilities is valuable given the more vulnerable population in these facilities and the higher use of antibiotics in these settings. Detection of antibiotic resistance genes using current laboratory PCR methods alone, however, is of questionable utility for public health action because antibiotic resistance can occur in both bacterial pathogens and commensal bacteria, which are carried without causing disease in most individuals. For example, several ESBL-conferring genes including bla_{CTX-M} are already commonly carried in human microbiomes (Woerther et al., 2013) and detected ubiquitously and in high levels in wastewater using PCR-based methods (Amos et al., 2014; Auguet et al., 2017; Rodriguez-Mozaz et al., 2015). Wastewater detection of rare antibiotic-resistant genes at a facility would likely trigger follow-up testing (e.g., selection by microbial culture, long-read genomic sequencing, proximity ligation sequencing) to determine whether the target antibiotic resistance genes are linked to pathogens. These approaches are difficult to integrate into the sample handling, laboratory analysis, and data analysis currently in place for routine national wastewater surveillance (Brown et al., 2021). Once antibiotic-resistant pathogens are confirmed at a facility, actions such as disinfection, individual clinical testing, contact prevention, and contact tracing could be implemented to limit its spread.

Periodic community-based wastewater surveillance for the rarer carbapenemases and colistin resistance genes would be useful to establish a baseline of which genes are present and could shed light on if or when organisms carrying these genes form reservoirs in wastewater systems. However, such periodic monitoring need only take place at a limited number of wastewater treatment plants across the United States to get useful data on baseline trends. Implementation at all NWSS community-based surveillance sites is likely to provide redundant baseline data that are not useful for public health action at the local scale.

OTHER POTENTIAL ENDEMIC TARGETS

Another target that has been publicly discussed for potential inclusion in NWSS national sampling is *Candida auris*. *C. auris* is a yeast and emerging pathogen with an extreme level of antimicrobial resistance and therefore of high public health significance. Most infections with *C. auris* to date have originated in a hospital setting, and current clinical screening approaches are recommended only for at-risk patients or residents. Relatively little is known about the distribution, reservoirs, or behavior of *C. auris* in the wastewater system (e.g., persistence, growth), although potential environmental reservoirs have been identified for other *Candida* species (Akinbobola et al., 2023; Stone et al., 2012). Therefore, interpretability of the data still needs to be established. Community-level wastewater surveillance of *C. auris* was first demonstrated during an ongoing outbreak in southern Nevada (Barber et al., 2023; Rossi et al., 2022) and has since been initiated in several other locations in Florida, California, and Arizona (e.g., Babler et al., 2023). Inclusion of *C. auris* in a wastewater surveillance panel to understand the breadth of distribution is understandable, but the actionability of community-level surveillance data may be limited. There are public health actions (e.g. contact prevention, contact tracing, environmental disinfection) that could be taken at long-term care facilities or hospitals if *C. auris* is detected. Barber et al. (2023) suggested that community-level wastewater surveillance may be useful in areas with no reported *C. auris* to spur additional screening at hospitals and long-term care facilities if a new community-level detection occurs. Overall, considering its healthcare-associated occurrence and the current uncertainty of its behavior in larger wastewater systems, facility-level rather than community-level surveillance may provide the best information to inform public health action, but continued exploration of the value of community-level versus facility-level surveillance still needs to be assessed. The ongoing surveillance by WastewaterSCAN for *C. auris* is expected to help close this gap.

Sexually transmitted infections (STIs) represent another potential opportunity for endemic wastewater surveillance. Additional information from wastewater on the occurrence of STIs, for which clinical case data are poor and slow to respond to outbreaks, could inform the allocation of resources to public health messaging campaigns and better inform clinicians. Although the analytical feasibility of wastewater surveillance has not been demonstrated for key targets like *Treponema palladium*, *Neisseria gonorrhea*, and *Chlamydia trachomatis*, molecular assays for their detection in clinical samples are readily available (Aboud et al., 2021; Tayoun et al., 2015).

CONSIDERATIONS WHEN REFINING
NWSS ENDEMIC TARGETS

Tradeoffs are involved when expanding wastewater surveillance targets in NWSS beyond a pilot scale. There are clear opportunities to increase the value of information from existing NWSS samples. However, there are additional analytical costs, the significance of which would depend on whether the new targets require different analytical concentration and extraction methods. Additional cost increases will be associated with data reporting, visualization, and analysis. In addition to needing to adapt existing local and national data visualization and analysis systems to include new targets, state and local public health authorities will need to manage, understand, and communicate the significance of the new target data in their communities. Public health jurisdictions have spent a considerable amount of time bringing wastewater surveillance online for SARS-CoV-2, including data analysis and public communication activities. While some states and localities actively use wastewater surveillance data to take public health action, others are still working to understand and communicate its value for decision making (see Chapter 4). Expansion of targets without a correlative increase in personnel time, training, and support tools may compound the burden on local public health. Another potential unintended consequence is loss of interest by some state and local public health jurisdictions due to a lack of understanding of why new targets were chosen and not finding them relevant to their local public health practice.

In light of budget uncertainty for the NWSS and potentially severe pending budget constraints (see Chapter 1), the recommendations for improving comparability and reducing variability in sampling and analysis and strengthening data analysis in the existing system (see Chapters 2, 3, and 4) are a higher priority than significantly expanding targets across NWSS sampling sites. By addressing these recommendations, the NWSS can ensure that public health agencies at local, state, and national scales can get the most information out of NWSS investments.

If budgets allow, an evidence-based, data-driven process that also considers local public health agency perspectives is needed prior to requiring additional targets in NWSS throughout the United States. Targets should only be added at all NWSS sites when specific uses for near-term or long-term public health action can be identified. Each of the targets discussed in this chapter meets one or more of the three criteria for new targets identified in the committee's Phase 1 report (Figure 5-1; NASEM, 2023), which suggests they are reasonable targets for consideration for nationwide surveillance. If funds are available, the committee supports the near-term addition of RSV and influenza, which meet the three NASEM (2023) criteria and can be processed using the same analytical methods as for SARS-CoV-2, reducing the additional analytical costs. For the other potential endemic targets discussed in this chapter, not all meet all three criteria, and more research or pilot testing may be needed to determine the feasibility and value of wastewater surveillance.

Prior to the inclusion of additional endemic targets at all NWSS sites, research should demonstrate that wastewater surveillance data can be reliably calibrated to public health outcomes of interest (NASEM, 2023). In some cases, this may be challenging as clinical data can be incomplete or nonexistent. Although one study has been conducted for correlations between adenovirus F40/41 and clinical sample positivity rates (Boehm et al., 2024), more studies are needed to understand the reliability of these trends to reflect infection in the community. Further, the bacterial enteric pathogens (STEC and *Campylobacter*) and antibiotic resistance gene targets do not yet have wastewater surveillance data that have been shown to reflect case burden or other health outcomes.

Approaches to address these research needs include both mechanistic and correlative approaches. Both have been applied to SARS-CoV-2 data and should not be considered mutually exclusive. For example, fecal shedding studies of SARS-CoV-2 during infection coupled with physical models of sewersheds demonstrated mechanistically the link between cases in a community and levels in wastewater (Prasek et al., 2022). Alternatively, many studies have identified strong correlations between COVID-19 cases in a community and wastewater concentrations (X. Li et al., 2023). For many of the expansion targets, good epidemiological data to relate to the wastewater surveillance data may be lacking, at least initially. Likewise, fecal shedding studies of most pathogens are sparse, limiting the mechanistic approach. Researchers have taken advantage of local outbreaks, such as with influenza A (Wolfe et al., 2022) and adenovirus 4 (Kazmer et al., 2024), to demonstrate correlations with wastewater. These outbreak periods resulted in higher clinical illness surveillance than during normal periods and thus provided a unique opportunity to study correlations between wastewater levels and cases. Prospective epidemiology studies could be used to validate measurements of community-wide burdens for comparison to wastewater data. Such studies would also begin to move the field forward toward using wastewater surveillance to estimate disease prevalence in addition to measuring trends.

A critical open question is to what degree wastewater surveillance of some of the individual targets would be able to inform public health action that reduces or prevents further spread and what is the value of this information for public health. Data from WastewaterSCAN may provide guidance on the value of additional targets for public health action.

The addition of targets may also have value for long-term public health action from the standpoint of understanding a disease, even when the short-term value of the data is limited due to the timing of wastewater surveillance data relative to disease dynamics. For example, a retrospective analysis of the spatial and temporal distribution of a target measured in wastewater in relation to limited annual case reports or outbreaks may improve the understanding of disease spread and inform future public health action. Such targets could be deemed worth adding at a pilot or national scale, particularly if they are added with minimal additional cost or sampling burden. However, such additions should be clearly communicated to states and localities as data that will be analyzed by researchers so that the burden of data analysis and interpretation is not perceived as resting on local public health agencies.

Much will continue to be learned about the value of wastewater surveillance beyond COVID-19 in the years ahead as new targets are incorporated and public health practitioners become more comfortable with the data. CDC should conduct a systematic review of any expanded targets 3–5 years after implementation to evaluate the value of the information provided for public health. This information can be used to further refine the wastewater surveillance targets for optimal public health benefit.

CONCLUSIONS AND RECOMMENDATIONS

The expansion of wastewater surveillance to include influenza and RSV in addition to SARS-CoV-2 is expected to provide useful public health information for minimal additional analytical costs, but more information is needed for several other targets prior to a decision to implement broadly across NWSS sites. The committee evaluated additional targets in active consideration by NWSS against the three criteria proposed in the Phase 1 report (NASEM, 2023): (1) the public health significance of the target, (2) analytical feasibility, and (3) the usefulness of community-level surveillance data to inform public health action. RSV, influenza, and SARS-CoV-2 clearly meet the three criteria and all of the proposed targets had public health significance. However, for other targets, data are not yet available to demonstrate that community-level wastewater surveillance data are correlated with health outcomes of interest or that the information is useful to inform near-term public health actions that can alter community infection dynamics. Ongoing data collection for several targets by WastewaterSCAN may fill this gap. Additional research or limited implementation supported by the NWSS Centers of Excellence can be used to resolve remaining uncertainties for proposed targets. Each pathogen target added has an accompanying cost to local and state public health agencies that collect that data associated with data analysis and interpretation. Therefore, the public health value of each new target should be clearly understood and communicated prior to nationwide implementation. Added targets should be reviewed after 3–5 years to determine the value and usefulness of the data for public health action. Under highly constrained budgets, the committee judges that improvements to data quality and comparability to be a higher near-term priority than target expansion.

The usefulness of routine wastewater surveillance for antibiotic resistance genes at the community (wastewater treatment plant) level is questionable because of limited ability to correlate the data with antibiotic resistance in clinically relevant pathogens. High priority antibiotic resistance phenotypes (such as carbapenem and vancomycin resistance) are encoded by multiple clusters of related genes and are present in wastewater in host-associated bacterial pathogens, a wide range of nonpathogenic bacteria found in humans, and other environmental reservoirs. Consequently, the laboratory methods currently used for wastewater surveillance are not always useful for detection of bacterial pathogens containing antibiotic resistance genes of interest. Approaches to link target antibiotic resistance genes to pathogens are difficult to integrate into the sample handling, laboratory analysis, and data analysis currently in place for routine national surveillance. Furthermore, the presence of antibiotic resistance genes from nonhuman sources, potential growth of organisms in biofilms within the wastewater systems, and the transfer and persistence of mobile resistance genes outside of a host confounds any interpretation at the community scale for public health action. The committee recommends that screening for antibiotic resistance genes focus on facility-level monitoring (e.g., hospitals, nursing homes) with wastewater treatment plant monitoring limited to specific needs, such as testing whether a high priority antibiotic resistance gene is widely present in the community. Additional culture-based analytical approaches would still be necessary at the facility level to confirm that the antibiotic resistance is associated with a pathogenic organism.

The following research and development needs should be addressed in the area of target identification:

- Explore the potential value of community-level wastewater surveillance data for adenovirus group F and norovirus for public health action.
- Determine the analytical feasibility and potential value of wastewater surveillance for STEC, *Campylobacter, Salmonella,* EVD68, and STIs, with an emphasis on determining the correlation between wastewater concentrations and health outcomes of interest and the extent to which these data are useful to support public health action.
- Understand the environmental reservoirs of antibiotic resistance genes to better gauge the potential value of wastewater surveillance at the community level.

6

Wastewater Surveillance for Emerging Pathogen Threats

Broadly, emerging pathogen threats fall into three categories. The first category includes known pathogens that have been identified as causing human disease in other countries but the risk for spread to the United States is unknown and potential for local containment is uncertain (e.g., SARS-CoV-2 at the outset of the global pandemic in early 2020; Mpox in 2023).[1] The second category involves pathogens present only in animals, either in the United States or internationally, with potential for spread into humans. Influenza viruses detected in poultry, swine, cattle, wild bird, or wild mammal populations exemplify this category. The third category consists of previously unknown pathogens with unknown properties that make preparation for an outbreak difficult—the "pathogen X" scenario.

The specific characteristics of wastewater surveillance for emerging pathogens in these three categories differ somewhat from the approaches described for endemic pathogens in Chapters 2–4 because, outside of an outbreak, they are not expected to be detected in U.S. wastewater samples. Surveillance for emerging (or re-emerging) threats presents a much higher level of uncertainty in terms of detection potential in wastewater, analytical sensitivity and specificity, and the distribution of temporal and spatial sampling needed to provide evidence and inform public health action on these rare but high-consequence targets. Surveillance will be triggered by key events, such as an outbreak in another region or detection of cases in the clinical setting (animal or human).

---

[1] See https://www.cdc.gov/poxvirus/mpox/outbreak/2023-drc.html.

In this chapter, the committee discusses potential uses of sentinel sites in a national wastewater surveillance system to address emerging and re-emerging pathogens. A sentinel site here refers to a location where enhanced or specific surveillance should take place because it represents a likely "front line" of entry to a larger community. The first section offers a vision for wastewater surveillance for emerging human pathogens that are previously known outside the United States or in animal populations. Sentinel sampling approaches, analytical methods, and specific needs for data analysis, visualization, and interpretation of wastewater surveillance data are discussed for these threats. In the final section of the chapter, the potential use of wastewater surveillance to address a "pathogen X" scenario and research and technology development opportunities associated with nontargeted detection are reviewed.

VISION FOR WASTEWATER SURVEILLANCE FOR KNOWN, EMERGING PATHOGEN THREATS

This section presents a vision for sentinel-site-based wastewater surveillance of emerging pathogen threats that are known to public health agencies. These include emerging human pathogens that may be limited to certain high-risk states (e.g., dengue virus in the southern United States) and those with epidemic or pandemic potential with serious consequences to public health that are known from prior disease outbreaks or detection outside the United States. Also included are diseases known to occur in animals with potential for human transmission.

Pathogens Emerging Outside the United States

The identification and reporting of the Omicron variant of SARS-CoV-2 in South Africa serves as a clear example of how internationally collaborative surveillance aided U.S. and global pandemic preparedness. The variant B.1.1.529 (Omicron) was first identified in South Africa and reported to the World Health Organization on November 24, 2021,[2] along with evidence of rapid spread within the country, thus providing an early warning to other nations. The first case was subsequently confirmed in the United States on December 1, 2021, and Omicron became the dominant variant by the end of the month (Iuliano et al., 2022). This advance warning allowed the U.S. surveillance systems, including wastewater surveillance, to initiate specific testing for B.1.1.529 and alerted hospital systems to take measures to preserve intensive care unit bed availability (Kirby et al., 2022). In retrospect,

---

[2] See https://www.who.int/news/item/26-11-2021-classification-of-omicron-(b.1.1.529)-sars-cov-2-variant-of-concern.

wastewater surveillance would have been similarly informative for SARS-CoV-1, a distinct coronavirus belonging to the same taxonomic grouping (Sarbecovirus) as SARS-CoV-2, which was first identified in 2003 as a cause of human morbidity and mortality outside the United States. The risk for spread of SARS-CoV-1 into the United States was unknown, but only syndromic surveillance was available with no population-based testing that would have been afforded by a national wastewater surveillance system.

Wastewater surveillance at sentinel sites could substantially enhance systematic surveillance for pandemic preparedness, including pathogens emerging outside the United States. Among the promising candidates for sentinel sites for routine surveillance are airports across the country that serve large numbers of international passengers and international mass gatherings and sporting events. Routine ongoing wastewater surveillance at these sites would provide baseline data before outbreaks and enable early detection of pathogen spread, supporting an effective outbreak response. If or when concerns are raised about a potential pandemic threat, this sentinel sampling can be intensified in terms of frequency and granularity, perhaps even targeting aircraft lavatory waste on arrival from specific countries with outbreaks, depending on the specific threat and potential public health actions. For example, wastewater surveillance for human cases of Middle East respiratory syndrome coronavirus (MERS-CoV) (Box 6-1) would focus on flights arriving from Middle Eastern countries where humans frequently come into contact with camelids, as well as other countries experiencing an outbreak of MERS. If airplane-specific data are collected, the results could be used for contact tracing or to encourage or require passengers to undergo follow-up testing or quarantine, depending on the threat. If pooled

---

BOX 6-1
Emergence and International Spread of MERS-CoV

Middle East respiratory syndrome coronavirus (MERS-CoV) emerged in Saudi Arabia, where it was initially detected in humans, with camels later identified as the animal host for zoonotic transmission to humans. Importantly, MERS-CoV infection has a higher case fatality rate, as compared to either SARS-CoV-1 or SARS-CoV-2. Although contact with camels was a major risk factor, direct human-to-human transmission also occurred, raising the risk for international spread due to global travel. International spread outside the Middle East was reported in 2018 in the U.K. and in South Korea, with exportation via human cases and localized epidemics. Wastewater surveillance at sentinel sites would be valuable in the case of a recurrence of MERS-CoV similar to that reported in 2018, given the high case fatality rate and the potential for onward human-to-human transmission (Milne-Price et al., 2014).

data from airplanes are collected, the data could be used to notify local and national agencies and clinicians of a new public health threat.

Similarly, the detection of an outbreak of a known but nonendemic pathogen could trigger localized or regional surveillance based on the understanding of specific risk factors. These pathogens are considered too rare to have value for routine monitoring throughout the National Wastewater Surveillance System (NWSS), but localized community-level wastewater surveillance may have strong utility once triggered by another data source, such as an increase in local community cases, hospitalizations, deaths, or other syndromic surveillance markers. Having a truly national system for wastewater surveillance would allow a rapid response, using the existing system for sample collection, processing, analysis, and reporting. The dengue virus outbreak in 2022–2023 is an example of this regional threat, based on distribution of the mosquito vector responsible for its transmission (Box 6-2). In addition, existing NWSS samples from affected regions could be analyzed for these additional targets until the pathogen outbreak is no longer seen as a significant threat. This approach is currently used informally by many jurisdictions (e.g., in response to local emergence/ outbreaks of polio, measles, hepatitis A, or Mpox). This type of flexibility was highlighted as a key characteristic in the NASEM (2023) vision of national wastewater surveillance. The committee notes that this targeted

---

BOX 6-2
Emergence and Localized Outbreak of
Dengue Virus in the United States

Dengue virus, transmitted by the mosquito species *Aedes aegypti*, is endemic in much of the subtropical and tropical regions worldwide. Notably, the prevalence of dengue infections has dramatically increased as the distribution of the mosquito vector has expanded. In the United States, dengue is endemic in Puerto Rico (as in much of the Caribbean) with 1,293 cases reported in 2023 and a current more severe outbreak resulting in an emergency declaration. While most cases detected in Florida are "imported" (i.e., infections acquired elsewhere), there is also evidence of local transmission. Subsequently, wastewater surveillance in Miami was found to be capable of detecting serotype 3 dengue virus in wastewater at a time when the same serotype was responsible for only 4.2 reported cases per 1 million population (Wolfe et al., 2024). These findings indicate that wastewater surveillance would be an effective tool for early seasonal spread in the Commonwealth of Puerto Rico and detection of spread within the vulnerable regions of the southern continental United States. Public health actions include both awareness of the public for individual mosquito control as well as community-based mosquito control.

"emergency" surveillance would likely require additional national, state, or municipal resources, but having a robust functioning national system for endemic pathogens (e.g., SARS-CoV-2) allows rapid deployment in response to an outbreak or high-level risk of such an outbreak, avoiding the time lag required to start a wastewater surveillance program where one does not exist.

Pathogens Emerging from Animal Sources

An estimated 75 percent of all recent emergent human pathogens originated in animal hosts (Taylor et al., 2001). These include those with direct animal-to-human transmission (e.g., rabies virus), transmission via an animal product (e.g., *Salmonella*), and transmission among humans after initially emerging from an animal host or hosts (e.g., influenza, MERS-CoV [see Box 6-1]). The majority of animal pathogens are most likely species- or genus-restricted and have limited, if any, risk for zoonotic transmission. Consequently, identifying useful targets for routine wastewater surveillance from among pathogens newly emerging from animal sources, in the absence of identified human infections, is challenging. Thus, wastewater surveillance of new or emerging pathogens with the potential for human transmission should be considered as an additional tool when justified based on data on infectious disease outbreaks in animals. National and state laboratories (e.g., the National Animal Health Laboratory Network) routinely investigate outbreaks of infectious diseases in the animal production sector to ensure a safe food supply in the United States and have the analytical capacity to detect pathogens in domesticated animals. Newly recognized or particularly rare animal pathogens are best investigated directly in livestock production surveillance programs, agricultural isolation facilities, and clinical settings where transmission dynamics and zoonotic potential can be investigated and disease reporting to relevant authorities should be routine.

Incorporation of animal pathogens into wastewater surveillance could be triggered by animal disease outbreaks with known or a high likelihood of risk for spread into domestic animal production and human populations in close contact with susceptible animals. As an example, H5N1 avian virus bird and mammal outbreaks represent events that should trigger considerations for wastewater surveillance, given the high risk for H5 influenza viruses to infect humans. The recent spread of H5N1 influenza A into dairy cows with transmission to farm workers reflects the highly adaptive and dynamic nature of influenza viruses and makes a case for ongoing vigilance for zoonotic viruses with high propensity for mutations (CDC, 2023a; Uyeki et al., 2024). The potential for detection of the influenza H5 gene in wastewater was demonstrated at three wastewater treatment plants with agricultural inputs in a state where H5N1 influenza was identified in dairy cattle (Wolfe et al., 2024b). Other avian influenza viruses with high probability of infecting humans, such as H7 and H9, would also be priority targets for sentinel-site-based wastewater surveillance in the event that outbreaks are observed in animal production facilities.

Identifying sentinel wastewater surveillance sites that could be ramped up in response to outbreaks would enable the development of an integrated animal and human surveillance system that complements clinical case detection. Sentinel sites would ideally be located in communities where high concentrations of people reside who work in animal production or processing. These sentinel sites should be identified in advance, with support from the U.S. Department of Agriculture (USDA), so that wastewater surveillance could be initiated rapidly when a disease with potential zoonotic transmission is detected in animals by animal health surveillance. In these settings, wastewater surveillance could enable early detection, assess rapidly changing outbreak dynamics, and inform effective combined responses that engage both animal and human health sectors.

SAMPLING FOR EMERGING PATHOGEN THREATS

In this section, the committee discusses sampling characteristics for emerging pathogen threats.

Sampling Design

A primary challenge for designing wastewater surveillance for emerging pathogen threats, including those that have been well characterized, is that the initial goal is to determine whether the pathogen is or is not present in the population—a binary outcome. Whereas a single positive test result can trigger additional testing, including repeat sampling and genetic sequencing to confirm the detection, a nondetection at a large wastewater treatment plant could mean the virus is present at a level that is currently beneath the detection limit. The significance of a nondetection is affected by the analytical detection threshold, the prevalence within the sampled population, the size of the population sampled, the probability that infected people will contribute waste to a sample, and the quantity of pathogen (or pathogen nucleic acid) shed into a waste stream Therefore, sentinel-based surveillance will enhance the predictive value of wastewater testing strategies, relative to surveillance at large wastewater treatment plants, by concentrating efforts on smaller at-risk populations where occurrence of emerging infections is more likely to be detected with current technology.

A sampling design for an emerging pathogen threat also needs to be developed with a clear vision for what actions will be taken if detection occurs. For example, if wastewater surveillance is conducted to detect a rare but high-consequence emerging pathogen from a single region, sampling of wastewater from incoming aircraft from that region could be conducted, but such granular data are most useful if actions will be taken to require quarantine or further testing of the passengers from planes with confirmed positive results. In contrast, if the public health goal is to inform local communities to prepare for a new emerging disease, sampling of triturators that pool waste from many planes may be more appropriate (and would reduce costs). In this chapter, the committee presents its vision for a sentinel surveillance program based on current understanding of emerging public health threats and useful actions that could be taken, but emerging pathogen surveillance ultimately requires flexibility to be successful. Necessary temporal and spatial resolution of sampling sites would be expected to evolve with changing assessments of public health threats, both nationally and internationally. Public health agencies' views on what actions they need to take regarding emerging pathogens under various scenarios may also evolve over time.

Optimized sampling for pandemic preparedness targets does not require routine surveillance at all locations. Doing so would be inefficient and jeopardize the sustainability of the surveillance system (as seen with ending of Project Biowatch in 2014). The following sections discuss sentinel sampling characteristics for known, emerging human pathogens and known emerging pathogens with zoonotic risk from animal sources.

Sampling Characteristics for Known Emerging Human Pathogens Sentinel Site Sampling Locations

Airplane and airport monitoring. In the year ending December 2023, 237 million airline passengers transited between the United States and other countries (USDOT, 2024). Airport-based, aircraft-based, and arriving traveler sentinel surveillance have been shown to have the greatest potential to rapidly detect the importation of recognized pathogens that are circulating outside the United States (Agrawal et al., 2022; J. Li et al., 2023; Wegrzyn et al., 2023). Wastewater sampling at airports can be conducted at a range of scales:

- At an airport-based wastewater treatment plant or downstream sewer line to sample the entire airport (including staff, travelers, and airplane waste),
- At an international terminal (including staff and travelers),
- At triturators that combine and process airplane lavatory waste from all incoming aircraft prior to release into the sewer system, and

- From individual planes when lavatory waste is emptied at the end of each route.

To address active known threats emerging from other countries and spread through human-to-human transmission, monitoring would most appropriately focus on aircraft arriving from international locations. Aircraft-based wastewater surveillance offers early detection of pathogen spread into the United States from regions where these pathogens have emerged. For aircraft-based sampling in the earliest phases of epidemics, long-haul flights entering the country are most productive and efficient, given the likelihood of passengers to use the toilet on the aircraft (Jones et al., 2023). Early research showed six of eight aircraft vessels had a positive SARS-CoV-2 detection in wastewater when only a single case on each flight was identified (Bivins et al., 2024). Ahmed et al. (2022) sampled long-haul flights arriving in Australia and reported a positive predictive value of 87.5 percent and a negative predictive value of 76.9 percent based on clinical detections of airline passengers during a subsequent 14-day quarantine. In contrast to other airport sampling, aircraft sampling is more granular and can be targeted toward pathogens of concern with specific countries of origin. (See Box 6-3 for a hypothetical example.) This surveillance approach

---

BOX 6-3
Hypothetical Example of Sentinel Airplane Monitoring:
Limiting Spread of SARS-CoV-1

Severe acute respiratory syndrome-coronavirus-1 (SARS-CoV-1) caused a severe respiratory illness first reported in Guangdong Province, China, in 2002. Although highly likely to have its origin in bats, the palm civet may have served as an intermediate host for zoonotic transmission to humans. The virus spread to 29 countries and resulted in 8,422 cases with a case fatality of approximately 11 percent (Chan-Yeung and Xu, 2003).

Consider a hypothetical situation in which SARS-CoV-1 has re-emerged in southeastern China. In response to this information, aircraft waste sampling is initiated on all direct flights from southeast China at several U.S. international airports and analyzed for SARS-CoV-1. It is found that waste samples obtained from a flight entering the United States 2 days ago are positive for SARS-CoV-1. Accordingly, epidemiologists obtain manifests for that flight. Passengers are contacted and asked to voluntarily provide samples for clinical testing, and all passengers are advised to voluntarily quarantine for 14 days. Two adults traveling together are found to be positive. This approach is in marked contrast to initiating contact tracing only after hospitalization, the traditional approach which imposes a significant lag time on response, thus increasing the likelihood of widespread transmission.

may also be useful for detection of pathogens that could be circulating in countries where there is inadequate surveillance and reporting to identify country-specific risk for pathogen importation into the United States. However, sampling of individual planes is staff intensive and costly and should be triggered only when there is a clearly identified threat and a defined public health response action.

Sampling at an airport triturator facility provides a composite sample limited to arriving aircraft (i.e., without addition of nontraveling airport personnel), can be automated, and has the least burden on airline and airport personnel. In a pilot program, the Centers for Disease Control and Prevention (CDC) has implemented surveillance using an automated sampler device at the San Francisco International Airport triturator.

To be able to respond in a timely manner, NWSS will need to pilot sentinel sampling approaches to meet different scenarios, so that the sampling strategies and uncertainties are well understood before the next public health emergency. Baseline data collection at these sentinel sites can be used to evaluate the sensitivity and specificity of this sentinel program in detecting outbreaks that are occurring in international locations. For example, information on SARS-CoV-2 variants through this baseline surveillance and additional pilot sampling efforts for individual long-haul international flights could be compared to data reported globally to evaluate capabilities for rapid and accurate detection of internationally imported cases. CDC is currently piloting wastewater surveillance in airplanes and airports and analyzing the results in comparison to individual voluntary passenger screening through its Traveler-Based Genomic Surveillance program and air sampling at airports (Tanne, 2023).[3] Meanwhile, other emerging technologies (e.g., airborne virus sampling; Ramuta et al., 2022) and existing approaches (Appiah et al., 2022) should continue to be assessed for use in international airports, airplanes, and other transportation centers, given their capacity to sample incoming travelers at a large scale and tailor testing to detect emerging pathogens prior to their spread in the community.

International event monitoring. In addition to airport- and aircraft-based surveillance, sentinel surveillance could include wastewater sampling in municipalities hosting multiday international events (e.g., sporting and entertainment events, conferences) to detect localized infectious disease transmission from an imported case or cases. Wastewater surveillance could be considered as part of the toolkit for early detection and monitoring for disease outbreaks at large events and could potentially complement bioterrorism monitoring (Elachola et al., 2016). Host cities could make wastewater monitoring part of their permitting and funding requirements for large

---

[3] See https://wwwnc.cdc.gov/travel/page/travel-genomic-surveillance.

events, connecting event planners with individuals and organizations that are already involved in the wastewater surveillance in the region.

Wastewater treatment plant monitoring. If analytical methods can detect extremely low levels of emerging pathogens or if high shedding rates occur for a target organism, existing wastewater surveillance samples from select cities in the United States could also serve as sentinel surveillance data. This would expand the population covered by sentinel-site monitoring without any additional sampling. However, public health actions facilitated by community-level wastewater surveillance data would differ from information gained from a specific flight. Also, if very few cases exist in a large city, false negatives are more likely to occur. Confidence limits for the presence of an emerging pathogen, if in fact it was present, could be computed to assess the feasibility of using a municipal wastewater treatment plant as a sentinel site for an emerging pathogen (see Box 6-4). Once a pathogen has been detected and is spreading within a community, emergency wastewater surveillance at the wastewater treatment plant scale can be used to monitor trends and potential recurrence in that locality and inform public health actions (Box 6-5).

BOX 6-4
Assessing Emerging Pathogen Detectability

Chen and Bibby (2023a) have described a modeling framework for evaluating the likelihood of detecting novel targets shed in feces, urine, or saliva in wastewater-based surveillance. Under their framework, a probabilistic model is used to relate analytical method sensitivity limits with levels of the target expected to be in wastewater. Distributions for parameters of shedding rates, wastewater per capita flow rates, and process limits of detection are populated based on a review of the literature, followed by a Monte Carlo simulation. Finally, a feasibility analysis is conducted to assess the minimum infectivity rate required for detection of the target by a method with a specific number of technical replicates and defined limit of detection. In a second paper, Chen and Bibby (2023b) developed a specific model for Zika virus using this approach to determine its utility as a wastewater surveillance target. Based on the output of their model, greater than one in a thousand people in a population would need to be shedding Zika virus to have a 50 percent chance of detection in the United States using the most sensitive methods evaluated, thus making community-level wastewater surveillance of this target impractical for early detection in non-endemic regions.

BOX 6-5
Emergency Wastewater Surveillance for Mpox

Mpox was initially rolled out as a wastewater surveillance target in response to the recent 2022 outbreak and proved to be remarkably sensitive (Adams et al., 2024; Wolfe et al., 2023b). Mpox is a rare viral infection that can cause a rash and flu-like symptoms. It has an extended incubation period (up to 3 weeks) during which an infected person can unknowingly transmit the disease. As a result, wastewater surveillance offered substantial lead time on clinical detections and enabled localities to mobilize public health resources, such as alerting clinicians and increased public health messaging, particularly toward at-risk communities, that encouraged prevention, testing, and vaccinations (Wolfe et al., 2023b). Because the outbreak has waned as of mid-2024, continued monitoring at sentinel sites with higher numbers of at-risk populations, with the flexibility to scale up quickly to national sampling as needed could save resources, rather than implementing nationwide.

Sampling Frequency for Emerging Human Pathogens

Sentinel surveillance at airports or other major ports of entry for new pandemic threats will be most useful for the first few days or weeks during the onset of an epidemic or an outbreak emerging in a new country or location, when findings can translate to action. The temporal sampling intensity for an emerging agent in the population should be based on the urgency and scale of the actions that might be taken if the emerging pathogen is detected. For example, monitoring for an emerging deadly virus with human-to-human transmission would merit much more intense sampling (e.g., individual aircraft level) than for a new, but mild illness.

Once a specific emerging pathogen becomes widespread in the population, sentinel monitoring for that pathogen at ports of entry is no longer needed. If the pathogen continues to pose a significant public health risk and wastewater surveillance provides useful information to support public health response, it could be added as an emergency target to existing or expanded wastewater surveillance in affected areas (Box 6-5) or, if useful, added to the NWSS core panel of endemic targets that are monitored across the nation.

Sampling for Pathogens Emerging from Animal Sources

Animal disease outbreak data can guide where to locate sentinel wastewater surveillance sites, although finding appropriate sites may be challenging because wastewater systems tend to underserve the rural areas where most intensive animal production occurs. Therefore, sewershed maps should be overlaid with locations where cattle, swine, and poultry production and slaughterhouses are located and/or large numbers of animal agricultural workers reside in order to identify potential sentinel sites. Such sites should be identified with assistance from the USDA and assessed in advance for the feasibility of wastewater surveillance so they can be rapidly activated in the event of animal outbreaks with high risk of zoonotic spillover. Although baseline data are less important when looking for emerging pathogens than for other pathogens, adding some such sites to NWSS for routine sampling may be beneficial to ensure that capacity is already built into the wastewater surveillance system for more intensive sentinel-site sampling when needed.

A major limitation of using wastewater surveillance for understanding the transmission of zoonotic pathogens is that current molecular detection methods in wastewater cannot distinguish between animal and human infections if there are sources of animal waste in the wastewater or presence of other materials containing zoonotic pathogens discharged into wastewater, such as milk. Ideally, sentinel sewered sites would be identified that are not likely to be confounded by animal waste inputs to maximize the specificity for detection of cases and outbreaks in humans. Sentinel sites could be tested for baseline levels of animal markers that could determine the extent of contamination at sites. Even for sites in which animal-based inputs are expected to be minimal, detection of animal pathogens in wastewater will require follow-up by testing methods optimized to distinguish animal infections from human infections (Fisher et al., 2015; Noble et al., 2003; Sinton et al., 1998). Triangulation of wastewater data with potential animal-based sources as well as active surveillance to assess the occurrence of clinical and subclinical cases in humans would constitute a coordinated and integrated approach to emerging pathogens from animal sources.

Biosafety Issues

As mentioned in Chapter 2, determination of appropriate biosafety protocols is needed in advance to ensure that the staff responsible for sampling and processing the samples have necessary protections in place to handle potential future targets and that laboratories with the appropriate biosafety level have the analytical capacity. Groups developing biosafety recommendations should include individuals with expertise in wastewater sampling and analysis (as distinct from clinical laboratories) as well as microbial risk. It is important to understand existing biosafety protections in conventional wastewater handling[4] and that detectable genetic signatures of emerging pathogens in wastewater do not necessarily represent viable, infectious agents.

ANALYTICAL METHODS FOR
KNOWN, EMERGING PATHOGENS

When analytical methods for known, emerging pathogens are applied, first and foremost, it is critical that the assays used to detect the pathogens are sensitive and specific. Pathogen-specific (targeted) analytical techniques for surveillance for known, emerging human and animal pathogens (including pathogens endemic outside of the United States) are used largely at universities and government agencies that have worked to detect pathogens where outbreaks have occurred to date. Reference genomes exist in public databases, and polymerase chain reaction (PCR) assays have been developed for clinical detection of the specific emerging pathogen. Thus, the molecular detection techniques used to identify these pathogens will be similar to that described for endemic pathogens in Chapter 3. However, the sensitivity and specificity of existing PCR assays designed for clinical samples need to be assessed for application to wastewater and the specific sentinel-site conditions. An example of how a clinical PCR assay has been adapted for wastewater monitoring is the use of the non-variola orthopox (Mpox) clinical PCR test, which now has been adapted for monitoring this pathogen in wastewater. CDC should invest in additional methods development to ensure that appropriate assays are available for emerging pathogens of pandemic potential and that these assays are validated in a range of wastewater samples. A formal advisory committee to NWSS could be valuable in shaping analytical method and assay development and providing rapid advice as needed in the realm of emerging pathogens. Furthermore, for emerging animal pathogens with zoonotic potential, collaboration and resource sharing with the USDA and U.S. Agency for International Development would reduce effort duplication and support data sharing.

Among zoonotic pathogens of particular concern for public health, coronaviruses and influenza viruses are known to be readily detected in wastewater (see Chapter 5), but there are fewer data on wastewater detection of zoonotic paramyxoviruses and flaviviruses. Studies on other high-risk pathogens would guide decisions on how best to implement wastewater-based surveillance at sentinel sites and focus efforts for further method development and refinement.

---

[4] See https://www.cdc.gov/global-water-sanitation-hygiene/about/workers_handlingwaste.html#cdc_generic_section_2-personal-protective-equipment-ppe.

Emerging pathogen targets of interest may be present in a sample at very low abundance, especially in wastewater samples with a larger contributing population that dilutes the sample. Therefore, methods with low detection levels and high specificity are particularly valuable to detect emerging targets while minimizing false negatives and false positives. As discussed in Chapter 3, digital PCR has been shown to be more sensitive with lower limits of detection for SARS-CoV-2 and is less likely to be impacted by the presence of inhibitors, which can cause falsely negative results (Ahmed et al., 2022a; Ciesielski et al., 2021). Quantitative PCR requires a standard curve, which can introduce variability if not performed meticulously. However, digital PCR equipment is more expensive. Ultimately, sentinel-site sample processing and analytical methods should be standardized, given the importance of comparable data across the nation when assessing emerging pathogens of pandemic threat.

Unlike with standard NWSS analytical methods for endemic pathogens, positive detections of emerging pathogens require particular scrutiny because it is possible that false positives can occur, and public health agencies will likely need confirmation that the laboratory analytical results are accurate before taking action. Laboratories that process sentinel-site samples should implement strict quality criteria and protocols, as discussed in Chapter 3, including consistent use of spike-in controls that assess nucleic acid extraction efficiency and assay sensitivity. In accordance with best practices, all negative results should be reported in light of the limits of detection for specific pathogens. Positive results should be individually inspected, with re-analysis of the sample and confirmatory sequencing. Quality control protocols for sentinel-site samples should be standardized so that all data are of the same laboratory quality. If something has not been detected before or is rarely detected, the laboratory should flag it for follow-up validation when reporting to the public health agency. In Chapter 3, trade-offs between sample processing and analysis speed, cost, and sensitivity were discussed for endemic pathogens, but for emerging pathogens, accuracy and sensitivity are the highest priorities. Given the extensive amount of work required to follow up on positive results and the potential public health implications of false negatives, investments that reduce detection limits while also improving specificity will save resources in the long run.

Although the planned sentinel surveillance assays are expected to be performed and reported in real time, circumstances may arise where it is advisable to retrospectively analyze archived samples to determine trends of newly detected pathogen signals. Therefore, all processed samples from sentinel sites should be archived for a minimum of 3 months to ensure that samples can be re-analyzed if data quality issues are raised. However, archiving for up to a year would be useful to confirm absence of detection prior to any pathogen emergence timeline and/or better refine timelines for outbreak emergence.

DATA ANALYSIS, INTERPRETATION, COMMUNICATION, AND INTERVENTION PLANNING FOR EMERGING PATHOGENS

Wastewater surveillance's key contribution to safeguarding public health is identifying when a new pathogen has entered the community so that public health authorities can quickly intervene. Therefore, the tools and strategies for information sharing, visualization, and data analysis for emerging pathogens in wastewater will need to be designed primarily for public health agencies rather than the general public.

In a national sentinel monitoring program, CDC should bear primary responsibility for standardizing protocols and conducting real-time analysis of the data, while sharing the data and interpretation with local public health agencies on a regular, pre-defined basis, regardless of whether or not a threat is detected. CDC should design tools and strategies for visualization and data analysis to evaluate potential pandemic threats, utilizing information on other detections and clinical data, including data from outside of the United States. As part of ongoing pandemic preparedness and response planning, CDC should prepare response action plans for a range of scenarios based on key factors, including its confidence level that the pathogen is detected, the timeliness of the information, and its understanding of the severity of associated health effects, expected duration of illness, spread mechanism, and potential interventions. These plans should include internal and external communication instructions and indicate which entity (CDC or local agency) is responsible for implementation, tracking, and reporting of intervention plan actions. CDC, potentially through the Centers of Excellence, should practice response action plan implementation with local public health agencies using tabletop exercises to ensure that localities are prepared.

To assist interagency coordination and make the best use of existing resources, wastewater surveillance should be included in the existing notifiable disease reporting system. State government (public health, agriculture agencies), national (CDC, USDA), and international programs (World Health Organization, World Organisation for Animal Health) for surveillance and reporting of notifiable human and animal diseases provide outstanding infrastructure including expertise, resources, and communication support. Including wastewater detections in this infrastructure will maximize public health actionability of this information.

EMERGING TECHNIQUES FOR FUTURE PUBLIC HEALTH MONITORING OF UNRECOGNIZED PATHOGENS

To date, validated laboratory assays that have been developed and used for diagnosis of infections in either humans or animals have been adapted for wastewater surveillance. However, syndromic surveillance can detect outbreaks caused by previously unknown pathogens for which no definitive laboratory or wastewater compatible test exists. These agents fall into two broad groupings: (1) variants of a known pathogen species or a "new" pathogen species or strains but within a known family (e.g., coronaviruses, orthomyxoviruses) and (2) truly novel pathogens. While clusters of human or animal infection due to an unknown pathogen are investigated, untargeted or semi-targeted methods can be used to detect and sequence these types of novel agents. Once "pathogen X" sequences are widely available, pathogen-specific assays (see Chapter 3) can be developed within days to weeks to detect the novel pathogen and shared broadly. Then, wastewater surveillance strategies can be designed to target these now known pathogens using more readily available analytical equipment, as discussed previously in this chapter (known, emerging pathogens). In this section, the state of technology for detection of unknown, emerging pathogens is discussed, followed by a review of the potential of these untargeted methods in the future of wastewater surveillance.

State of Technology for Semi-targeted and Untargeted Analytical Methods

The majority of wastewater surveillance efforts have been focused on a handful of known, high-priority pathogens, but, in the future, it is possible that wastewater surveillance will broaden to monitor the emergence and evolution of unrecognized pathogens and other important epidemiological transitions. The committee envisions that two broad categories of approaches not in active use right now could be used to surveil for these types of agents: a semi-targeted and a fully untargeted approach.

Semi-targeted Methods

A semi-targeted approach can include methods such as amplicon sequencing, microarray, or hybrid capture and sequencing. Amplicon sequencing (Figure 6-1), which is currently among the most widely applied semi-targeted methods, involves PCR amplifying a specific DNA region of a target genome using primers, or short DNA sequences, that are complementary to highly conserved regions of the target DNA. An example of

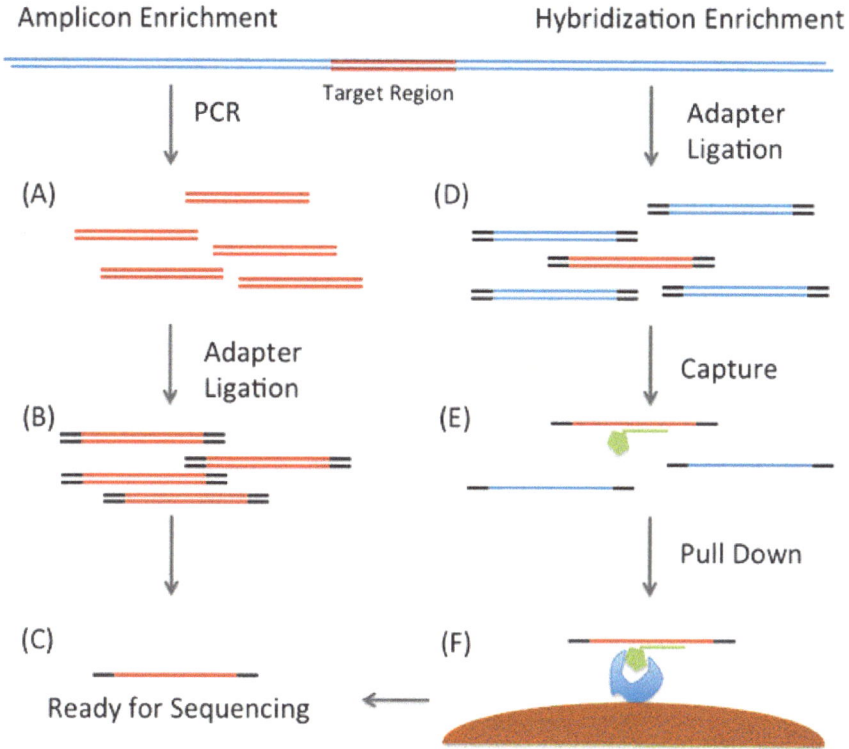

FIGURE 6-1 Two semi-targeted sequence enrichment methods. Amplicon enrichment uses primers to isolate a sequence of interest. In hybridization enrichment, the RNA or DNA is sheared into smaller fragments, and a capture probe (or bait sequence) binds with complementary sequences and is then isolated with magnetic beads.
SOURCE: https://www.researchgate.net/figure/A-comparison-of-two-popular-sequence-enrichment-methods-A-For-amplicon-enrichment-PCR_fig1_273781301.

amplicon sequencing is 16S rRNA gene sequencing, where primers are generated to bind to highly conserved regions of the 16S rRNA gene, which is a "marker gene" in bacteria and other prokaryotes. Once amplicons are generated, the intervening region is amplified and then sequenced. The intervening region is variable among different organisms, and thus the amplified sequence, or amplicon, can be compared to reference genomes which then will provide information about the composition of prokaryotic organisms within the samples. In addition to use for sequencing of prokaryotic communities, other types of amplicons can be generated. For example, these types of approaches have proven quite useful in the identification of and surveillance for SARS-CoV-2 variants in the past. In this case, variable regions of the SARS-CoV-2 genome are amplified using primers against highly conserved regions of the genome. These types of methods provide insight into emerging variants and are more cost-effective than fully untargeted methods, which are outlined below.

In addition to amplicon sequencing, a similar but technologically distinct approach is to use a hybrid capture (see Figure 6-1). In this approach, a single-stranded nucleic acid sequence that is complementary to a pathogen or pathogens of interest is developed. All nucleic acid sequences that are complementary (i.e., similar) enough to that "bait" sequence are bound by it. This approach allows for imperfect complementarity, and thus novel variants that are somewhat related to known targets can be recovered. The sequences that are "captured" by the bait are then sequenced and analyzed (Nasir et al., 2020). Microarrays are similar to hybrid capture except that hybridization is assessed directly, typically through fluorescent tags; sequencing is not performed. Microarrays provide a fast and inexpensive way to identify differences between closely related genomes (Gresham et al., 2008).

Untargeted Methods

While the semi-targeted approaches outlined above can be useful in identifying novel targets that are related to known targets, they are less useful for totally novel or "unknown unknowns." Such targets may be viral, prokaryotic, or eukaryotic in nature. To detect such targets, assuming they are organisms with DNA or RNA as their genetic material as opposed to protein-based infectious agents (prions), untargeted approaches can be used. These methods provide information on the totality of DNA and RNA sequences that are within a sample. Such a sample can be a bulk metagenomic sample or viral particle enrichment. Interpretation of these data in complex sample types such as wastewater, in which there are likely thousands or more different microbes in addition to other types of nucleic acid from sources such as foodstuffs, is much less straightforward than for clinical samples.

Untargeted analysis methods for wastewater might fall into one of two major categories. In the first category, efforts might be made to identify the novel target or pathogen of interest in a "reference-free" manner. This type of approach could build on well-established methods that have been pioneered in the study of environmental and host-associated microbiomes (e.g., shotgun whole genome sequencing for DNA or total RNA sequencing; see Figure 6-2), in which the genome is broken up into small pieces, which are then assembled using computational algorithms into larger genomic fragments. This type of approach, which is akin to putting together the pieces

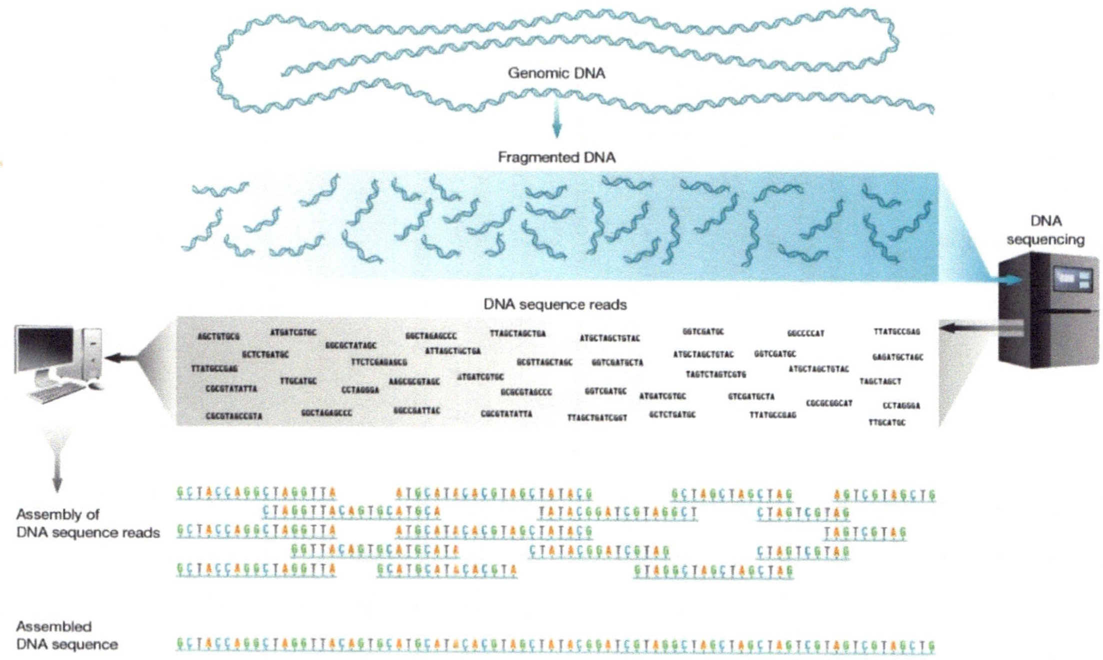

FIGURE 6-2 Shotgun DNA sequencing involves breaking up the genome into small fragments that are individually sequenced and then analyzed to reconstruct as much of the original genome as possible.
SOURCE: https://www.genome.gov/genetics-glossary/Shotgun-Sequencing.

of a jigsaw puzzle from a mixture of puzzle pieces, enables the identification of novel organisms or targets that might be present in a sample (Parks et al., 2017; Tyson et al., 2004). When such a sample is compared to a reference library of known organisms, novel agents could be discovered. Indeed, these types of approaches have enabled the assembly and surveillance of important agricultural pathogens, such as the tomato brown rugose fruit virus, a recently emerged pathogen of nightshade plants (Natarajan et al., 2023; Salem et al., 2015).

In the second category of untargeted analysis, shotgun metagenomic data can be queried in a "reference-based" manner. Here, untargeted metagenomic data are compared to a large, well-curated database of available and relevant reference sequences using read-based or marker-based approaches. Such approaches could identify the presence of a novel variant of a known pathogen, such as mutated versions of the mpox virus. Alternatively, this could serve as a way to query increasing and decreasing abundances of novel, emerging candidate antimicrobial resistance genes that have some level of relatedness to known genes.

Excellent approaches exist for the types of analysis outlined in both reference-free and reference-based strategies, and with modern computing capabilities, many of these analyses can be carried out quickly and with relative ease. All methods require there to be adequate abundance of the organism to be detected within the given sample. The number of sequences per sample ("sequencing depth") collected determines how sensitive a given assay is, and deeper coverage improves specificity substantially because the ability to distinguish a pathogen from its close relatives becomes greater. Untargeted analysis of wastewater may necessitate very deep sequencing to detect signals from pathogens that may be rare or poorly abundant in the samples. All in all, these data can provide information that can guide the development and execution of more targeted and quantitative assays that follow up on these initial screens and subsequently allow for the development of targeted and cheap detection methods for specific pathogens discovered during this untargeted discovery phase.

Although untargeted sequencing methods can be tuned to be exquisitely sensitive, there can be trade-offs between sensitivity and specificity. This can be particularly challenging when an emerging pathogen or target of interest shares substantial genomic sequence homology with harmless, prevalent, and abundant nonpathogens. Rapid read-based methods for data analysis cannot in principle distinguish closely related organisms. With current technology, to differentiate between two closely related organisms can require additional detailed and sometimes customized data analysis that may involve applying so-called "metagenotyping computational tools"

(Zhao et al., 2022) to deep shotgun sequencing data. These types of processes require knowledgeable scientists and large computer resources to carry out.

These technical and workforce issues currently limit the scalability of assay interpretation from a public health application perspective, but many opportunities exist in the research space. While expensive, and therefore not routine, generation of metagenomic data from wastewater will enable both prospective and retrospective evaluation of known, emerging, and novel pathogens, and this may help inform future public health applications. For example, total RNA or DNA sequencing of historically banked samples might enable identification of emergence or re-emergence of pathogens, such as a bird flu or *Salmonella enterica* outbreaks. By mining existing data or samples from pre-outbreak time periods, researchers could possibly evaluate the cost-effectiveness of such approaches for sensitively and specifically detecting future outbreaks.

It is possible that other signals in wastewater that are secondary to the pathogen of interest might be altered in the presence of a pathogen, and in these cases, future analytical approaches may focus on the discovery of these secondary signals as opposed to rare pathogen signals. However, development and application of these types of approaches will require additional analytical advancements, likely aided by the rapid emergence of artificial intelligence–based data analysis tools. Overall, while untargeted methods hold great promise, because of the limitations enumerated above, they have yet to enter the mainstream.

LOOKING AHEAD

Although semi- and untargeted methods may not be ready to roll out on a broad and national level at present, as future molecular and analytical approaches evolve and are refined, it is expected that such data will be an important part of future surveillance efforts. Indeed, large-scale efforts to collect longitudinal biological data in a well-curated manner (for example, collection of protein structures in the Protein Data Bank[5]) have enabled great advances in machine learning–based protein structure prediction (Jumper et al., 2021). Few, if any, could have anticipated that having such protein structure data would eventually lead to machine learning–driven computer programs that can accurately and quickly predict the protein structures of nearly any amino acid sequence. Thus, the committee anticipates that continued close communication between wastewater scientists and engineers, microbiologists, health care researchers, epidemiologists, and data scientists will be critical in this next phase of innovation.

---

[5] See https://www.rcsb.org/.

There are several ways in which modern artificial intelligence approaches may enhance the effectiveness and utility of wastewater surveillance for emerging pathogens. First, machine-learning approaches excel at automated pattern recognition and thus may be optimally positioned to identify patterns and anomalies in large datasets. For example, new variants of SARS-CoV-2 could be readily identified from large datasets by identifying newly present short RNA sequences, where parts of the sequence have similarities to known SARS-CoV-2 but specific regions are different. Second, once an adequate set of wastewater surveillance data and outcomes is developed, predictive models can be developed, which might provide advance warning of upcoming shifts in disease incidence and prevalence. Finally, with advances in computing capabilities and artificial intelligence algorithms, it is possible to incorporate a variety of highly diverse data types to inform integrated datasets that might further improve predictive models. Although current investment in artificial intelligence related research is primarily through the National Institutes of Health (NIH) and the National Science Foundation (NSF), CDC and its NWSS Centers of Excellence should periodically evaluate applicability of modern machine-learning approaches to wastewater surveillance.

A carefully considered investment in this realm may enable early detection of targets or pathogens that are so-called black swans—events that come as a surprise and have a major effect (Velappan et al., 2022). With advancements in data analytics, wastewater surveillance may allow scientists to follow the totality of the sequence data (as a combined and very rich source of information on both pathogens and the microbiome response to pathogens) over time. Changes in the patterns of the composition of the sequence data that are beyond typical variance could be determined by advanced machine learning methods. These deviations from patterns could then be triangulated with other available data, such as clinical syndrome information or climate information, to identify possible evidence of emerging epidemiological shifts.

All in all, while trade-offs exist in making investments in these types of future-focused efforts versus more immediate or near-term surveillance efforts, an arm of wastewater-based surveillance research and development that looks to the future and adapts to the strengths of emerging technologies and analytical approaches is sage. In the near term, the types of efforts described in this section may be information-gathering exercises and are unlikely to trigger specific public health actions, but with the learning that is gained over time, they may transform into leading indicators of emerging pathogens, and thus may help prepare our public health system for specific actions.

CONCLUSIONS AND RECOMMENDATIONS

The committee's Phase 1 report (NASEM, 2023) recommended strategic incorporation of sentinel sites in the NWSS to allow early detection of emerging pathogen threats. Ideally, a wastewater surveillance system for emerging threats could identify pathogens as they enter the country. Importantly, the routine surveillance provided by the NWSS allows rapid emergency response to a disease outbreak, which may be national (e.g., an emerging SARS-CoV-2 variant), regional (e.g., dengue virus), or limited to high-risk settings (e.g. Influenza H5N1 in dairy communities). These detections would enable timely public health actions, such as targeted therapies or recommendations regarding behaviors (e.g., limiting contact with others) that could mitigate the spread of and adverse outcomes associated with the disease. This chapter discusses specific characteristics of wastewater surveillance at sentinel sites for emerging pathogens and for emergency outbreak response.

International traveler–based wastewater surveillance at airports serving large numbers of arriving international passengers would provide critical sentinel surveillance sites for emerging pathogens. With current technology, sample collection at triturators would allow the most focused and cost-effective sampling of incoming aircraft without additional burden on the airlines and airline personnel. Several (<10) of the largest international airports in the United States should be selected to provide a geographically diverse set of sentinel sites. Sentinel-site samples should be processed and analyzed in a rapid, reliable, and consistent manner to ease data comparison and interpretation and support a timely response. Such sentinel sites would enhance potential local and national response strategies, ranging from early warning to additional testing and quarantine of passengers, depending on the significance of the threat and resources invested. CDC can leverage resources developed for traveler-based programs. CDC should ensure that this sentinel monitoring strategy has clear links to public health action, with plans and protocols for local and national response based on the pathogen detected. CDC should also periodically review the program so that the sentinel strategy stays abreast of technology development, including ongoing assessment of alternative strategies such as airborne pathogen monitoring.

CDC should identify additional, uniquely targeted sentinel sites to provide surveillance for human infections emerging from animal sources. As zoonotic pathogens can emerge from intensified livestock production, CDC should ensure coverage of select representative at-risk communities working in intensive animal production and slaughtering, particularly avian species and swine due to their role in influenza A evolution and transmission. Additional testing may be necessary to distinguish animal infections from human infections.

Temporary community-level wastewater surveillance could provide valuable information on international introductions associated with mass gathering events and localized epidemics and inform public health response. Large-scale public events (e.g., Olympic games, World Cup) where tens or hundreds of thousands of travelers are expected to congregate pose risk for accidental introduction and spread of pathogens, especially if drawing in crowds from international locations for several days. Incorporation of wastewater surveillance in advance event planning and permitting would help ensure readiness for epidemic and pandemic monitoring as needed. Likewise, highly localized outbreaks may merit temporary infectious disease surveillance at the community scale in affected areas.

CDC should bear the primary responsibility for conducting real-time analysis of data from NWSS sentinel sites, rapidly sharing verified data with local, state, and tribal public health agencies and developing a rapid-response plan. Real-time analysis and interpretation of emerging pathogen data from sentinel monitoring sites requires context and situation updates from coordinated international, national, and state public health (and potentially animal health) authorities, which is beyond the reach of most local public health agencies. CDC should develop laboratory and agency guidance and protocols to ensure rapid re-analysis and verification of emerging pathogen detections and ancillary data. Additionally, it should develop guidance for local, state, and tribal agencies on how to respond to positive detections, including additional data collection, interventions, and communication.

Wastewater surveillance should be linked with notifiable disease reporting systems to enhance existing infrastructure for interagency communication. To achieve this, pathogens classified as notifiable diseases that are detected in wastewater should be reported within existing local, national, and international disease reporting systems. These programs for surveillance and reporting of notifiable human and animal diseases provide resources including expertise and communication support. Data on detection of notifiable pathogens in wastewater should be seamlessly shared between animal and human health agencies to help local, state, national, and international health agencies track and respond to emerging outbreaks.

Research and technical development in partnership with academic labs that specialize in pathogen detection will help augment and advance wastewater surveillance efforts for use in monitoring emerging pathogens. Specifically, the following research needs are high priority:

- **Ongoing assessment of the suitability of wastewater surveillance for newly emerging pathogens.** Research that assesses whether an emerging pathogen is shed into wastewater by infected persons and can be detected in wastewater, and whether such data add value beyond existing testing and surveillance methods, will help identify pathogens for further method development.

- **Continued development and improvement of analytical methods for suspected emerging agents of concern in wastewater,** including enrichment approaches, detection thresholds and detection confirmation criteria. Many of the known emerging pathogen threats have available analytical assays, but these analytical methods have not been optimized for wastewater. Additional work on suspected agents of concern is needed to ensure that appropriate wastewater analysis methods are available when needed and their sensitivity and specificity understood across a range of wastewater matrix characteristics.
- **Development of systems for rapid sentinel-site data analysis and integration** with other disease reporting systems.
- **Continued refinement and optimization of the siting of emerging pathogen surveillance.** As technologies and analytical approaches improve, leading to increased sensitivity of detection, surveillance of rare and emerging threats may become feasible at the wastewater treatment plant level. Ultimately, envisioned public health response strategies will dictate the best scale for sentinel-site sampling.

Research to adapt and apply nontargeted sequencing methods along with advanced statistical and machine learning–based analysis approaches to wastewater surveillance are expected to be fruitful for expanding future public health benefits. Target-agnostic methods, such as high-throughput short- and long-read DNA sequencing, are rapidly advancing but the approach in wastewater surveillance is currently costly and not routinely applied. Target-agnostic methods, when paired with creative analytical approaches and artificial intelligence, have the potential to provide information on population-level shifts and detect changes in targets of interest, including emerging and unknown pathogens and antimicrobial resistance genes. Such data, if collected in a structured manner and alongside complementary types of data, such as public health and vaccination data, might facilitate the use of machine learning–based approaches to develop predictive models based on these rich data types. This remains an exploratory research space with investment primarily from NIH and NSF, but given the rapid advances in artificial intelligence and machine learning–based analytics, it is expected to be a promising and potentially useful avenue for future investment and CDC should periodically review application to wastewater surveillance.

References

Aboud, L., Y. Xu, E. P. F. Chow, T. Wi, R. Baggaley, M. B. Mello, C. K. Fairley, and J. J. Ong. 2021. Diagnostic accuracy of pooling urine, anorectal, and oropharyngeal specimens for the detection of *Chlamydia trachomatis* and *Neisseria gonorrhoeae*: A systematic review and meta-analysis. *BMC Medicine* 19:285. https://doi.org/10.1186/s12916-021-02160-9 (accessed May 3, 2024).

Adams, C., A. Kirby, M. Bias, A. Riser, K. K. Wong, J. W. Mercante, and H. Reese. 2024. Detecting Mpox cases through wastewater surveillance—United States, August 2022–May 2023. *Morbidity and Mortality Weekly Report* 73(2):37–43. https://www.cdc.gov/mmwr/volumes/73/wr/pdfs/mm7302a3-H.pdf (accessed April 1, 2024).

Agrawal, S., L. Orschler, S. Tavazzi, R. Greither, B. M. Gawlik, and S. Lackner. 2022. Genome sequencing of wastewater confirms the arrival of the SARS-CoV-2 omicron variant at Frankfurt Airport but limited spread in the City of Frankfurt, Germany, in November 2021. *Microbiology Resource Announcements* 11(2). https://doi.org/10.1128/mra.01229-21 (accessed May 3, 2024).

Ahmed, W., A. Bivins, P. M. Bertsch, K. Bibby, P. M. Choi, K. Karkas, P. Gyawali, K. A. Hamilton, E. Haramoto, M. Kitajima, S. L. Simpson, S. Tondukar, K. V. Thomas, and J. F. Mueller. 2020. Surveillance of SARS-CoV-2 RNA in wastewater: Methods optimization and quality control are crucial for generating reliable public health information. *Current Opinion in Environmental Science & Health* 17:82–93. https://doi.org/10.1016/j.coesh.2020.09.003 (accessed May 3, 2024).

Ahmed, W., A. Bivins, S. L. Simpson, P. M. Bertsch, J. Ehret, I. Hosegood, S. S. Metcalfe, W. J. M. Smith, K. V. Thomas, J. Tynan, and J. F. Mueller. 2022a. Wastewater surveillance demonstrates high predictive value for COVID-19 infection on board repatriation flights to Australia. *Environment International* 158:106938 (accessed May 3, 2024).

Ahmed, W., W. J. M. Smith, S. Metcalfe, G. Jackson, P. M. Choi, M. Morrison, D. Field, P. Gyawali, A. Bivins, K. Bibby, and S. L. Simpson. 2022b. Comparison of RT-qPCR and RT-dPCR platforms for the trace detection of SARS-CoV-2 RNA in wastewater. *American Chemical Society Publications* 2(11):1871–1880. https://doi.org/10.1021/acsestwater.1c00387 (accessed May 3, 2024).

Ahmed, W., et al. 2022c. Minimizing errors in RT-PCR detection and quantification of SARS-CoV-2 RNA for wastewater surveillance. *Science of the Total Environment* 805:149877.

Ai, Y., A. Davis, D. Jones, S. Lemeshow, H. Tu, F. He, P. Re, X. Pan, Z. Bohrerova, and J. Lee. 2021. Wastewater SARS-CoV-2 monitoring as a community-level COVID-19 trend tracker and variants in Ohio, United States. *Science of the Total Environment* 801:149757.

Akinbobola, A. B., R. Kean, S. M. A. Hanifi, and R. S. Quilliam. 2023. Environmental reservoirs of the drug-resistant pathogenic yeast *Candida auris*. *PLoS Pathogens* 19(4):1011268. https://doi.org/10.1371/journal.ppat.1011268 (accessed May 3, 2024).

Allayeh, A. K., S. A. Al-Daim, N. Ahmed, M. El-Gayar, and A. Mostafa. 2022. Isolation and genotyping of adenoviruses from wastewater and diarrheal samples in Egypt from 2016 to 2020. *Viruses* 14(10):2192. https://doi.org/10.3390/v14102192 (accessed May 3, 2024).

Ammerman, M. L., S. Mullapudi, J. Gilbert, K. Figueroa, F. P. N. Cruz, K. M. Bakker, M. C. Eisenberg, B. Foxman, and K. R. Wigginton. 2024. Norovirus GII wastewater monitoring for epidemiological surveillance. *PLoS Water* 3(1):e0000198. https://doi.org/10.1371/journal.pwat.0000198 (accessed May 3, 2024).

Amos, G. C. A., P. M. Hawkey, W. H. Gaze, and E. M. Ellington. 2014. Wastewater effluent contributes to the dissemination of CTX-M-15 in the natural environment. *Journal of Antimicrobial Chemotherapy* 69(7):1785–1791. https://doi.org/10.1093/jac/dku079 (accessed November 20, 2024).

Appiah, G., T. Smith, R. Wegrzyn, R. C. Morfino, S. Guadliardo, S. Milford, A. T. Walker, E. T. Ernst, W. W. Darrow, S. L. Li, T. Aichele, A. Rothstein, B. Rome, D. MacCannell, G. Woronoff, K. Robinson, D. Dai, B. Girinathan, A. Hicks, B. Cosca, A. Plocik, B. Simen, L. Moriarty, M. S. Cetron, and C. R. Friedman. 2022. The impact of traveler-based genomic surveillance on SARS-CoV-2 variant detection in arriving international air travelers—United States, November 29, 2021–April 24, 2022. *Open Forum Infectious Diseases* 9(Suppl 2). https://doi.org/10.1093/ofid/ofac492.087 (accessed May 6, 2024).

Arora, M., J. Moser, H. Phadke, A. A. Basha, and S. L. Spencer. 2017. Endogenous replication stress in mother cells leads to quiescence of daughter cells. *Cell Reports* 19(7):1351–1364. https://doi.org/10.1016/j.celrep.2017.04.055 (accessed May 6, 2024).

Arts, P. J., J. D. Kelly, C. M. Midgley, K. Anglin, S. Lu, G. R. Abedi, R. Andino, K. M. Bakker, B. Banman, A. B. Boehm, and M. Briggs-Hagen. 2023. Longitudinal and quantitative fecal shedding dynamics of SARS-CoV-2, pepper mild mottle virus, and crAssphage. *Msphere* 8(4):e00132-23. https://doi.org/10.1128/msphere.00132-23 (accessed May 6, 2024).

APHL (Association of Public Health Laboratories). 2022. *SARS-CoV-2 wastewater surveillance testing guide for public health laboratories*. Association of Public Health Laboratories. https://www.aphl.org/aboutAPHL/publications/Documents/EH-2022-SARSCoV2-Wastewater-Surveillance-Testing-Guide.pdf (accessed May 3, 2024).

APHL. 2024. *National trends in wastewater surveillance 2023 survey report*. https://www.aphl.org/aboutAPHL/publications/Documents/EH-2023-Wastewater-Survey.pdf (accessed June 26, 2024)

Auguet, O. T., M. Pijuan, C. M. Borrego, S. Rodriguez-Mozaz, X. Triado-Margarit, S. V. D. Giustina, and O. Gutierrez. 2017. Sewers as potential reservoirs of antibiotic resistance. *Science of the Total Environment* 605–606:1047–1054. https://doi.org/10.1016/j.scitotenv.2017.06.153 (accessed May 6, 2024).

Babler, K., M. Sharkey, S. Arenas, A. Amirali, C. Beaver, S. Comerford, K. Goodman, G. Grills, M. Holung, E. Kobetz, J. Laine, W. Lamar, C. Mason, D. Pronty, B. Reding, S. Schurer, N. S. Solle, M. Stevenson, D. Vidovic, H. Solo-Gabriele, and B. Shukla. 2023. Detection of the clinically persistent, pathogenic yeast spp. Candida auris from hospital and municipal wastewater in Miami-Dade County, Florida. *Science of the Total Environment* 898:165459. https://doi.org/10.1016/j.scitotenv.2023.165459 (accessed May 6, 2024).

Barber, C., K. Crank, K. Papp, G. K. Innes, B. W. Schmitz, J. Chavez, A. Rossi, and D. Gerrity. 2023. Community-scale wastewater surveillance of *Candida auris* during an ongoing outbreak in southern Nevada. *Environmental Science & Technology | American Chemical Society Publications* 57(4):1755–1763. https://doi.org/10.1021/acs.est.2c07763 (accessed May 6, 2024).

Barry-Jester, A. M. 2022. Health officials see bright future in poop surveillance. KFF Health News-formerly KHN. https://kffhealthnews.org/news/article/sewage-surveillance-tracking-covid-infectious-disease-modesto-california/ (accessed June 14, 2024).

Beattie, R.E., A.D. Blackwood, T. Clerkin, C. Dinga, and R.T. Noble. 2022. Evaluating the impact of sample storage, handling, and technical ability on the decay and recovery of SARS-CoV-2 in wastewater. *PLOS ONE* 17(6):e0270659. https://doi.org/10.1371/journal.pone.0270659 (accessed July 12, 2024).

Bivins, A., et al. 2020. Wastewater-based epidemiology: Global collaborative to maximize contributions in the fight against COVID-19. *Environmental Science & Technology | American Chemical Society Publications* 54(13):7754–7757. https://doi.org/10.1021/acs.est.0c02388 (accessed May 6, 2024).

Bivins, A., D. North, Z. Wu, M. Shaffer, W. Ahmed, and K. Bibby. 2021. Within- and between-day variability of SARS-CoV-2 RNA in municipal wastewater during periods of varying COVID-19 prevalence and positivity. *Environmental Science & Technology Water| American Chemical Society Publications* 1(9):2097–2108. https://doi.org/10.1021/acsestwater.1c00178 (accessed May 6, 2024).

Bivins, A., D. Kaya, W. Ahmed, J. Brown, C. Butler, J. Greaves, R. Leal, K. Maas, G. Rao, S. Sherchan, D. Sills, R. Sinclair, R. T. Wheeler, and C. Mansfeldt. 2022. Passive sampling to scale wastewater surveillance of infectious disease: Lessons learned from COVID-19. *Science of the Total Environment* 835:155347. https://doi.org/10.1016/j.scitotenv.2022.155347 (accessed May 6, 2024).

Bivins, A., A. Franklin, S. Simpson, and W. Ahmed. 2023. The lavatory lens: Tracking the global movement of pathogens via aircraft wastewater. *Critical Reviews in Environmental Science and Technology* 54(4):1–21. https://doi.org/10.1080/10643389.2023.2239129 (accessed November 20, 2024).

Blaser, M.J. 2004. Bacteria and diseases of unknown cause: Hemolytic-uremic syndrome. *Journal of Infectious Diseases* 189(3):552–563. https://doi.org/10.1086/381129 (accessed May 6, 2024).

Boehm, A. B., B. Hughes, D. Duong, V. Chan-Herur, A. Buchman, M. K. Wolfe, and B. J. White. 2023a. Wastewater concentrations of human influenza, metapneumovirus, parainfluenza, respiratory syncytial virus, rhinovirus, and seasonal coronavirus nucleic-acids during the COVID-19 pandemic: A surveillance study. *The Lancet Microbe* 4(5):e340–e348. https://doi.org/10.1016/s2666-5247(22)00386-x (accessed May 6, 2024).

Boehm, A., M. K. Wolfe, B. J. White, B. Hughes, and D. Duong. 2023b. Two years of longitudinal measurements of human adenovirus group F, norovirus GI and GII, rotavirus, enterovirus, enterovirus D68, hepatitis A virus, *Candida auris*, and West Nile virus nucleic acids in wastewater solids: A retrospective study at two wastewater treatment plants. *MedRxiv*. https://doi.org/10.1101/2023.08.22.23294424 (accessed May 6, 2024).

Boehm, A. B., M. K. Wolfe, B. J. White, B. Hughes, D. Duong, N. Banaei, and A. Bidwell. 2023c. Human norovirus (HuNoV) GII RNA in wastewater solids at 145 United States wastewater treatment plants: Comparison to positivity rates of clinical specimens and modeled estimates of HuNoV GII shedders. *Journal of Exposure Science & Environmental Epidemiology*. https://doi.org/10.1038/s41370-023-00592-4 (accessed May 6, 2024).

Boehm, A. B., D. A. Wadford, A. Chen, T. Padilla, C. Wright, L. Moua, T. Bullick, M. Salas, C. Morales, C. A. Glaser, D. J. Vugia, A. T. Yu, B. Hughes, D. Duong, B. J. White, and M. K. Wolfe. 2023d. Trends of enterovirus D68 concentrations in wastewater, California, USA, February 2021–April 2023. *Emerging Infectious Diseases* 29(11):2362. https://doi.org/10.3201/eid2911.231080 (accessed May 6, 2024).

Boehm, A. B., B. Shelden, D. Duong, N. Banaei, B. J. White, and M. K. Wolfe. 2024. A retrospective longitudinal study of adenovirus group F, norovirus GI and GII, rotavirus, and enterovirus nucleic acids in wastewater solids at two wastewater treatment plants: Solid-liquid partitioning and relation to clinical testing data. *mSphere* 9(3):e00736-23. https://doi.org/10.1128/msphere.00736-23 (accessed May 6, 2024).

Borchardt, M.A., A.B. Boehm, M. Salit, S.K. Spencer, K.R. Wigginton, and R.T. Noble. 2021. The Environmental Microbiology Minimum Information (EMMI) Guidelines: qPCR and dPCR quality and reporting for environmental microbiology. *Environmental Science & Technology* 55(15):10210–10223. https://doi.org/10.1021/acs.est.1c01767 (accessed July 12, 2024).

Breulmann, M., R. Kallies, K. Bernhard, A. Gasch, R. A. Muller, H. Harms, A. Chatzinotas, and M. van Afferden. 2023. A long-term passive sampling approach for wastewater-based monitoring of SARS-CoV-2 in Leipzig, Germany. *Science of the Total Environment* 887:164143. https://doi.org/10.1016/j.scitotenv.2023.164143 (accessed May 9, 2024).

Brouwer, A. F., J. N. S. Eisenberg, C. D. Pomeroy, L. M. Shulman, M. Hindiyeh, Y. Manor, I. Grotto, J. S. Koopman, and M. C. Eisenberg. 2018. Epidemiology of the silent polio outbreak in Rahat, Israel, based on modeling of environmental surveillance data. *Proceedings of the National Academy of Sciences* 115(45):E10625–E10633. https://doi.org/10.1073/pnas.1808798115 (accessed May 6, 2024).

Brown, C. L., I. M. Keenum, D. Dai, L. Zhang, P. J. Vikesland, and A. Pruden. 2021. Critical evaluation of short, long, and hybrid assembly for contextual analysis of antibiotic resistance genes in complex environmental metagenomes. *Scientific Reports* 11(1):3753. https://doi.org/10.1038/s41598-021-83081-8 (accessed May 6, 2024).

Bushnell, G., F. Mitrani-Gold, and L. M. Mundy. 2013. Emergence of New Delhi metallo-β-lactamase type 1-producing Enterobacteriaceae and non-Enterobacteriaceae: Global case detection and bacterial surveillance. *International Journal of Infectious Diseases* 17(5):e325–e333. https://doi.org/10.1016/j.ijid.2012.11.025 (accessed November 20, 2024).

Bustin, S.A., V. Benes, J. A. Garson, J. Hellemans, J. Huggett, M. Kubista, R. Mueller, T. Nolan, M. W. Pfaffl, G. L. Shipley, J. Vandesompele, and C. T. Wittwer. 2009. The MIQE guidelines: Minimum information for publication of quantitative real-time PCR experiments. *Clinical Chemistry* 55(4):611–622. https://doi.org/10.1373/clinchem.2008.112797 (accessed July 12, 2024).

Casanova, L., W. A. Rutala, D. J. Weber, and M. D. Sobsey. 2009. Survival of surrogate coronaviruses in water. *Water Research* 43(7):1893–1898. https://doi.org/10.1016/j.watres.2009.02.002 (accessed November 20, 2024).

CDC (Centers for Disease Control and Prevention). 2023a. *Technical report: Highly pathogenic avian influenza A(H5N1) viruses.* National Center for Immunization and Respiratory Diseases. https://www.cdc.gov/flu/avianflu/spotlights/2022-2023/h5n1-technical-report_december.htm (accessed May 9, 2024).

CDC. 2023b. *Wastewater surveillance testing methods.* National Wastewater Surveillance System. https://www.cdc.gov/nwss/testing.html (accessed May 9, 2024).

CDC. 2023c. *Press release: CDC announces $262M funding to support National Network for Outbreak Response and Disease Modeling.* September 22. https://www.cdc.gov/media/releases/2023/p0922-disease-modeling.html (accessed May 9, 2024).

CDC. 2023d. *Developing a wastewater surveillance sampling strategy.* National Wastewater Surveillance System. https://www.cdc.gov/nwss/sampling.html (accessed May 9, 2024).

CDC. 2023e. *Public health interpretation and use of wastewater surveillance data.* https://www.cdc.gov/nwss/interpretation.html (accessed June 29, 2024).

CDC. 2023f. *Wastewater surveillance data reporting and analytics.* https://www.cdc.gov/nwss/reporting.html (accessed June 29, 2024).

Chan, E. M., L. C. Kennedy, M. K. Wolfe, and A. B. Boehm. 2023. Identifying trends in SARS-CoV-2 RNA in wastewater to infer changing COVID-19 incidence: Effect of sampling frequency. *PLOS Water* 2(4):e0000088. https://doi.org/10.1371/journal.pwat.0000088 (accessed May 9, 2024).

Chan, P. K. S. 2002. Outbreak of avian influenza A (H5N1) virus infection in Hong Kong in 1997. *Clinical Infectious Diseases* 34(2):S58–S64. https://doi.org/10.1086/338820 (accessed May 9, 2024).

Chan-Yeung, M., and R. H. Xu. 2003. SARS: epidemiology. *Respirology* 8:S9–S14. https://doi.org/10.1046/j.1440-1843.2003.00518.x (accessed July 24, 2024).

Chen, W., and K. Bibby. 2023a. Making waves: Establishing a modeling framework to evaluate novel targets for wastewater-based surveillance. *Water Research* 245:120573.

Chen, W., and K. Bibby. 2023b. A model-based framework to assess the feasibility of monitoring zika virus with wastewater-based epidemiology. *ACS ES&T Water* 3(4):1071-1081.

Chik, A. H., M. B. Glier, M. Servos, C. S. Mangat, X. L. Pang, Y. qiu, P. M. D'Aoust, J. B. Burnet, R. Delatolla, S. Dorner, Q. Geng, J. P. Giesy Jr., R. M. McKay, M. R. Mulvey, N. Prystajecky, N. Srikanthan, Y. Xie, B. Conant, and S. E. Hrudey. 2021. Comparison of approaches to quantify SARS-CoV-2 in wastewater using RT-qPCR: results and implications from a collaborative inter-laboratory study in Canada. *Journal of Environmental Sciences* 107:218-229. https://doi.org/10.1016/j.jes.2021.01.029 (accessed July 24, 2024).

Chopra, A., A. Rodriguez, B. A. Prakash, R. Raskar, and T. Kingsley. 2023. Using neural networks to calibrate agent based models enables improved regional evidence for vaccine strategy and policy. *Vaccine* 41(48):7067–7071. https://doi.org/10.1016/j.vaccine.2023.08.060 (accessed May 9, 2024).

Ciannella, S., C. González-Fernández, and J. Gomez-Pastora. 2023. Recent progress on wastewater-based epidemiology for COVID-19 surveillance: A systematic review of analytical procedures and epidemiological modeling. *Science of the Total Environment* 878:162953.

Ciesielski, M., D. Blackwood, T. Clerkin, R. Gonzales, H. Thompson, A. Larson, and R. Noble. 2021. Assessing sensitivity and reproducibility of RT-ddPCR and RT-qPCR for the quantification of SARS-CoV-2 in wastewater. *Journal of Virological Methods* 297:114230. https://doi.org/10.1016/j.jviromet.2021.114230 (accessed May 9, 2024).

Colman, E., P. Holme, H. Sayama, and C. Gershenson. 2019. Efficient sentinel surveillance strategies for preventing epidemics on networks. *PLoS Computational Biology* 15(11):e1007517. https://doi.org/10.1371/journal.pcbi.1007517 (accessed May 9, 2024).

Crank, K., K. Papp, C. Barber, P. Wang, A. Bivins, and D. Gerrity. 2023. Correspondence on The Environmental Microbiology Minimum Information (EMMI) guidelines: qPCR and dPCR quality and reporting for environmental microbiology. *Environmental Science & Technology* 57(48):20448–20449. https://www.ncbi.nlm.nih.gov/pmc/articles/PMC10702426/ (accessed May 9, 2024).

Curtis, K., D. Keeling, K. Yetka, A. Larson, and R. Gonzalez. 2020. Wastewater SARS-CoV-2 RNA concentration and loading variability from grab and 24-hour composite samples. *MedRxiv.* https://doi.org/10.1101/2020.07.10.20150607 (accessed May 9, 2024).

Cutrupi, F., M. Rossi, M. Cadonna, E. Poznanski, S. Manara, M. Postinghel, G. Palumbi, M. Bellisomi, E. Nicosia, G. Allaria, L. Dondero, C. Veneri, P. Mancini, G. Bonanno Ferraro, G. Rosa, E. Suffredini, P. Foladori, and E. Grasselli. 2023. Evaluation of concentration procedures, sample pre-treatment, and storage condition for the detection of SARS-CoV-2 in wastewater. *Environmental Science and Pollution Research International* 30(48):106660–106670. https://doi.org/10.1007/s11356-023-29696-y (accessed July 12, 2024).

Daza-Torres, M. L., J. C. Montesinos-Lopez, C. Herrera, Y. E. Garcia, C. C. Naughton, H. N. Bischel, and M. Nuno. 2024. Optimizing spatial distribution of wastewater-based disease surveillance to advance health equity. *MedRxiv.* https://doi.org/10.1101/2024.05.02.24306777 (accessed June 24, 2024).

DeJonge, P. M., C. Adams, I. Pray, M. K. Schussman, R. B. Fahney, M. Shafer, D. S. Antkiewicz, and A. Roguet. 2023. Wastewater surveillance data as a complement to emergency department visit data for tracking incidence of influenza A and respiratory syncytial virus—Wisconsin, August 2022–March 2023. *Morbidity and Mortality Weekly Report* 72(37):1005–1009. https://doi.org/10.15585/mmwr.mm7237a2 (accessed May 9, 2024).

Dewey-Mattia, D., K. Maikonda, A. J. Hall, M. E. Wise, and S. J. Crowe. 2018. Surveillance for foodborne disease outbreaks—United States, 2009–2015. *Morbidity and Mortality Weekly Report* 67(10):1–11. https://doi.org/10.15585/mmwr.ss6710a1 (accessed May 9, 2024).

Dobis, E. A., T. Krumel, J. Cromartie, K. L. Thomas (Conley), A. Sanders, and R. Ortiz. 2012. *Rural America at a Glance: 2021 Edition.* U.S. Department of Agriculture Economic Research Service (EIB-230):18. https://www.ers.usda.gov/webdocs/publications/102576/eib-230.pdf?v=1920.3 (accessed May 9, 2024).

Dorélien, A. M., A. Simon, S. Hagge, K. T. Call, E. Enns, and S. Kulasingam. 2020. Minnesota social contacts and mixing patterns survey with implications for modelling of infectious disease transmission and control. *Survey Practice* 13(1). https://doi.org/10.29115/SP-2020-0007 (accessed May 9, 2024).

Drake, J. M., A. Handel, E. Marty, E. B. O'Dea, T. O'Sullivan, G. Righi, and A. T. Tredennick. 2023. A data-driven semi-parametric model of SARS-CoV-2 transmission in the United States. *PLoS Computational Biology* 19(11):e1011610. https://doi.org/10.1371/journal.pcbi.1011610 (accessed May 9, 2024).

Duvallet, C., F. Wu, K. A. McElroy, M. Imakaev, N. Endo, A. Xiao, J. Zhang, R. Floyd-O'Sullivan, M. M. Powell, S. Mendola, S. T. Wilson, F. Cruz, T. Melman, C. L. Sathyanarayana, S. W. Olsen, T. B. Erickson, N. Ghaeli, P. Chai, E. J. Alm, and M. Matus. 2022. Nationwide trends in COVID-19 cases and SARS-CoV-2 RNA wastewater concentrations in the United States. *ACS ES&T Water* 2(11):1899–1909. https://doi.org/10.1021/acsestwater.1c00434 (accessed May 9, 2024).

Elachola, H., E. Gozzer, J. Zhuo, S. Sow, R. Kattan, S. Mimesh, J. Al-Tawfiq, M. Al-Sultan, and Z. Memish. 2016. Mass gatherings: A one-stop opportunity to complement global disease surveillance. *Journal of Health Specialties* 4(3):178–185.

Environmental Protection Agency. 2023. *Wastewater sampling.* Athens, GA: Laboratory Services and Applied Science Division. http://www.epa.gov/sites/default/files/2017-07/documents/wastewater_sampling306_af.r4.pdf (accessed May 9, 2024).

Erster, O., I. Bar-Or, V. Levy, R. Shatzman-Steuerman, D. Sofer, L. Weiss, R. Vasserman, I. S. Fratty, K. Kestin, M. Elul, N. Levi, R. Alkrenawi, E. Mendelson, M. Mandelboim, and M. Weil. 2022. Monitoring of enterovirus D68 outbreak in Israel by a parallel clinical and wastewater based surveillance. *Viruses* 14(5):1010. https://doi.org/10.3390/v14051010 (accessed May 9, 2024).

Federal Task Force on Combating Antibiotic-Resistant Bacteria. 2020. *National action plan for combatting antibiotic-resistant bacteria.* https://aspe.hhs.gov/sites/default/files/migrated_legacy_files//196436/CARB-National-Action-Plan-2020-2025.pdf (accessed June 26, 2024).

Feng, S., A. Roguet, J. S. McClary-Gutierrez, R. J. Newton, N. Kloczko, J. G. Meiman, and S. L. McLellan. 2021. Evaluation of sampling, analysis, and normalization methods for SARS-CoV-2 concentrations in wastewater to assess COVID-19 burdens in Wisconsin communities. *ACS ES&T Water* 1(8):1955–1965. https://doi.org/10.1021/acsestwater.1c00160 (accessed May 9, 2024).

Fisher, J. C., A. M. Eren, H. C. Green, O. C. Shanks, H. G. Morrison, J. H. Vineis, M. L. Sogin, and S. L. McLellen. 2015. Comparison of sewage and animal fecal microbiomes by using oligotyping reveals potential human fecal indicators in multiple taxonomic groups. *Applied and Environmental Microbiology* 81(20):7023–7033. https://doi.org/10.1128/aem.01524-15 (accessed May 9, 2024).

Fung, B., A. Gopez, V. Servellita, S. Arevalo, C. Ho, A. Deucher, E. Thornborrow, C. Chiu, and S. Miller. 2020. Direct comparison of SARS-CoV-2 analytical limits of detection across seven molecular assays. *Journal of Clinical Microbiology* 58(9). https://doi.org/10.1128/jcm.01535-20 (accessed May 9, 2024).

George, A. L., D. Kaya, B. A. Layton, K. Bailey, S. Mansell, C. Kelly, K. J. Williamson, and T. S. Radneicki. 2022. Impact of sampling type, frequency, and scale of the collection system on SARS-CoV-2 quantification fidelity. *Environmental Science & Technology Letters* 9(2):160–165. https://doi.org/10.1021/acs.estlett.1c00882 (accessed May 9, 2024).

Ghebremedhin, B. 2014. Human adenovirus: Viral pathogen with increasing importance. *European Journal of Microbiology and Immunology* 4(1):26–33. https://doi.org/10.1556/eujmi.4.2014.1.2 (accessed May 9, 2024).

Godlewska, K., P. Stepnowski, and M. Paszkiewicz. 2020. Pollutant analysis using passive samplers: Principles, sorbents, calibration and applications. A review. *Environmental Chemistry Letters* 19(1):465–520. https://doi.org/10.1007/s10311-020-01079-6 (accessed May 9, 2024).

Graham, K. E., S. K. Loeb, M. K. Wolfe, D. Catoe, N. Sinnott-Armstrong, S. Kim, K. M. Yamahara, L. M. Sassoubre, L. M. M. Grijalva, L. Roldan, Hernandez, K. Langenfeld, K. R. Wigginton, and A. B. Boehm. 2020. SARS-CoV-2 RNA in wastewater settled solids is associated with COVID-19 cases in a large urban sewershed. *Environmental Science & Technology* 55(1):488–498. https://doi.org/10.1021/acs.est.0c06191 (accessed May 9, 2024).

Gresham, D., M. J. Dunham, and D. Botstein. 2008. Comparing whole genomes using DNA microarrays. *Nature Reviews Genetics* 9(4):291–302. https://doi.org/10.1038/nrg2335 (accessed May 9, 2024).

Habtewold, J., D. McCarthy, E. McBean, I. Law, L. Goodridge, M. Habash, and H. M. Murphy. 2022. Passive sampling, a practical method for wastewater-based surveillance of SARS-CoV-2. *Environmental Research* 204(Pt B):112058. https://doi.org/10.1016/j.envres.2021.112058 (accessed May 9, 2024).

Hackenberger, D., H. Imtiaz, A. R. Raphenya, B. P. Alcock, H. N. Poinar, G. D. Wright, and A. G. McArthur. 2024. CARPDM: Cost-effective antibiotic resistome profiling of metagenomic samples using targeted enrichment. *bioRxiv*. https://doi.org/10.1101/2024.03.27.587061 (accessed May 10, 2024).

Hart, O. E., and R. U. Halden. 2020. Modeling wastewater temperature and attenuation of sewage-borne biomarkers globally. *Water Research* 172:115473. https://doi.org/10.1016/j.watres.2020.115473 (accessed May 10, 2024).

Hassard, F., T. R. Smith, A. B. Boehm, S. Nolan, O. O'Mara, M. Di Cesare, and D. Graham. 2022. Wastewater surveillance for rapid identification of infectious diseases in prisons. *The Lancet Microbe* 3(8):e556–e557. https://doi.org/10.1016/S2666-5247(22)00154-9 (accessed May 10, 2024).

Hayes, E. K., A. K. Stoddart, and G. A. Gagnon. 2022. Adsorption of SARS-CoV-2 onto granular activated carbon (GAC) in wastewater: Implications for improvements in passive sampling. *Science of the Total Environment* 847:157548 https://doi.org/10.1016/j.scitotenv.2022.157548 (accessed May 10, 2024).

Hayes, E. K., C. L. Sweeney, L. E. Anderson, B. Li, G. B. Erjavec, M. T. Gouthro, W. H. KrKosek, A. K. Stoddart, and G. A. Gagnon. 2021. A novel passive sampling approach for SARS-CoV-2 in wastewater in a Canadian province with low prevalence of COVID-19. *Environmental Science: Water Research & Technology* 7(9):1576–1586. https://doi.org/10.1039/d1ew00207d (accessed May 10, 2024).

Heß, S., D. Kneis, T. Österlund, B. Li, E. Kristiansson, and T. U. Berendonk. 2019. Sewage from airplanes exhibits high abundance and diversity of antibiotic resistance genes. *Environmental Science & Technology* 53(23):13898–13905. https://doi.org/10.1021/acs. est.9b03236 (accessed May 10, 2024).

Hjelmsø, M. H., M. Hellmér, X. Fernandez-Cassi, N. Timoneda, O. Lukjancenko, M. Seidel, D. Elsässer, F. M. Aarestrup, C. Löfström, S. Bofill-Mas, J. F. Abril, R. Girones, and A. C. Schultz. 2017. Evaluation of methods for the concentration and extraction of viruses from sewage in the context of metagenomic sequencing. *PloS One* 12(1):e0170199. https://doi.org/10.1371/journal.pone.0170199 (accessed July 24, 2024).

Hewitt, J., S. Trowsdale, B. A. Armstrong, J. R. Chapman, K. M. Carter, D. M. Croucher, C. R. Trent, R. E. Sim, and B. J. Gilpin. 2022. Sensitivity of wastewater-based epidemiology for detection of SARS-CoV-2 RNA in a low prevalence setting. *Water Research* 211:118032. https://doi.org/10.1016/j.watres.2021.118032 (accessed May 10, 2024).

HHS (U.S. Department of Health and Human Services). 2020. *National action plan for combating antibiotic-resistant bacteria, 2020–2025.* Office of the Assistant Secretary for Planning and Evaluation: Office of Science and Data Policy. https://aspe.hhs.gov/reports/national-action-plan-combating-antibiotic-resistant-bacteria-2020-2025 (accessed May 10, 2024).

Holst, M. M., J. Person, W. Jennings, R. M. Welsh, M. J. Focazio, P. M. Bradley, W. B. Schill, A. E. Kirby, and Z. A. Marsh. 2022. Rapid implementation of high-frequency wastewater surveillance of SARS-CoV-2. *ACS ES&T Water* 2(11):2201–2210. https://doi.org/10.1021/acsestwater.2c00094 (accessed May 10, 2024).

Hopkins, L., D. Persse, K. Caton, K. Ensor, R. Schneider, C. McCall, and L. B. Stadler. 2023. Citywide wastewater SARS-CoV-2 levels strongly correlated with multiple disease surveillance indicators and outcomes over three COVID-19 waves. *Science of the Total Environment* 855:158967. https://doi.org/10.1016/j.scitotenv.2022.158967 (accessed May 10, 2024).

Huge, B. J., D. North, C. B. Mousseau, K. Bibby, N. J. Dovichi, and M. M. Champion. 2022. Comparison of RT-dPCR and RT-qPCR and the effects of freeze–thaw cycle and glycine release buffer for wastewater SARS-CoV-2 analysis. *Scientific Reports* 12:20641. https://doi.org/10.1038/s41598-022-25187-1 (accessed May 10, 2024).

Huggett, J. F., C. A. Foy, V. Benes, K. Emslie, J. A. Garson, R. Haynes, J. Hellemans, M. Kubista, R. D. Mueller, T. Nolan, M. W. Pfaffl, G. L. Shipley, J. Vandesompele, C. T. Wittwer, and S. A. Bustin. 2013. The digital MIQE guidelines: Minimum information for publication of quantitative digital PCR experiments. *Clinical Chemistry* 59(6):892–902. https://doi.org/10.1373/clinchem.2013.206375 (accessed July 12, 2024).

Hughes, B., D. Duong, B. J. White, K. R. Wigginton, E. M. G. Chan, M. K. Wolfe, and A. B. Boehm. 2022. Respiratory syncytial virus (RSV) RNA in wastewater settled solids reflects RSV clinical positivity rates. *Environmental Science and Technology Letters* 9(2):173–187. https://doi.org/10.1021/acs.estlett.1c00963 (accessed May 10, 2024).

Hughes, H. E., O. Edeghere, S. J. O'Brien, R. Vivancos, and A. J. Elliot. 2020. Emergency department syndromic surveillance systems: A systematic review. *BMC Public Health* 20(1891):1–15. https://doi.org/10.1186/s12889-020-09949-y (accessed May 10, 2024).

Huston, P., V. L. Edge, and E. Bernier. 2019. Reaping the benefits of open data in public health. *Canada Communicable Disease Report* 45(10):252–256. https://doi.org/10.14745/ccdr. v45i10a01 (accessed May 10, 2024).

Ingram, D. D., and S. J. Franco. 2013. NCHS urban–rural classification scheme for counties. National Center for Health Statistics. *Vital and Health Statistics* 2(166). https://www.cdc.gov/nchs/data/series/sr_02/sr02_166.pdf (accessed May 10, 2024).

IOM (Institute of Medicine). 2015. *Sharing clinical trial data: Maximizing benefits, minimizing risk.* Washington, DC: The National Academies Press. https://doi.org/10.17226/18998 (accessed July 12, 2024).

Islam, G., A. Gedge, L. Linda-Jacabo, A. Kirkwood, D. Simmons, and J-P. Desaulniers. 2022. Pasteurization, storage conditions and viral concentration methods influence RT-qPCR detection of SARS-CoV-2 RNA in wastewater. *Science of the Total Environment* 821: 153228.

Iuliano, A. D., et al. 2022. Trends in disease severity and health care utilization during the early omicron variant period compared with previous SARS-CoV-2 high transmission periods—United States, December 2020–January 2022. *Morbidity and Mortality Weekly Report* 71(4):146–152. https://doi.org/10.15585/mmwr.mm7104e4 (accessed May 10, 2024).

Jobling, K., M. Quintela-Beluja, F. Hassard, P. Adamou, A. Blackburn, S. McIntyre-Nolan, J. L. Romalde, M. Di Cesare, and D. W. Graham. 2024. Comparison of gene targets and sampling regimes for SARS-CoV-2 quantification for wastewater epidemiology in UK prisons. *Journal of Water and Health* 22(1):64–76. https://doi.org/10.2166/wh.2023.093 (accessed May 10, 2024).

Johnson, M. 2022. *CDC launches public COVID-19 wastewater surveillance dashboard.* Genome Web. https://www.genomeweb.com/covid-19/cdc-launches-public-covid-19-wastewater-surveillance-dashboard (accessed May 10, 2024).

Jones, G. M., E. Busby, J. A. Garson, P. R. Grant, E. Nastouli, A. S. Devonshire, and A. S. Whale. 2016. Digital PCR dynamic range is approaching that of real-time quantitative PCR. *Biomolecular Detection and Quantification* 10:31–33. https://doi.org/10.1016/j.bdq.2016.10.001 (accessed May 10, 2024).

Jones, D. L., J. M. Rhymes, M. J. Wade, J. L. Kevill, S. K. Malham, J. M. S. Grimsley, C. Rimmer, A. J. Weightman, and K. Farkas. 2023. Suitability of aircraft wastewater for pathogen detection and public health surveillance. *Science of the Total Environment* 856(Pt 2):159162. https://doi.org/10.1016/j.scitotenv.2022.159162 (accessed May 10, 2024).

Joung, M. J., C. S. Mangat, E. M. Mejia, A. Nagasawa, A. Nichani, C. Perez-Iratxeta, S. W. Peterson, and D. Champredon. 2023. Coupling wastewater-based epidemiological surveillance and modelling of SARS-CoV-2/COVID-19: Practical applications at the Public Health Agency of Canada. *Canada Communicable Disease Report* 49(5):166–174. https://doi.org/10.14745%2Fccdr.v49i05a01 (accessed May 10, 2024).

Jothikumar, N., T. L. Cromeans, V. R. Hill, X. Lu, M. D. Sobsey, and D. D. Erdman. 2005. Quantitative real-time PCR assays for detection of human adenoviruses and identification of serotypes 40 and 41. *Applied and Environmental Microbiology* 71(6):3131–3136. https://doi.org/10.1128/aem.71.6.3131-3136.2005 (accessed May 10, 2024).

Jumper, J., et al. 2021. Highly accurate protein structure prediction with AlphaFold. *Nature* 596(7873):583–589. https://www.nature.com/articles/s41586-021-03819-2 (accessed May 10, 2024).

Kazmer, K. R., M. L. Ammerman, E. A. Edwards, M. C. Eisenberg, J. Gilbert, J. P. Montgomery, V. M. Pierce, J. B. Weinberg, and K. R. Wigginton. 2024. Respiratory human adenovirus outbreak captured in wastewater surveillance. *medRxiv*. https://doi.org/10.1101/2024.06.15.24308982 (accessed July 11, 2024).

Kim, S., et al. 2022. SARS-CoV-2 RNA is enriched by orders of magnitude in primary settled solids relative to liquid wastewater at publicly owned treatment works. *Environmental Science: Water Research & Technology* 8(4):757–770. https://doi.org/10.1039/D1EW00826A (accessed May 10, 2024).

Kirby, A. E., et al. 2022. Notes from the field: Early evidence of the SARS-CoV-2 B.1.1.529 (omicron) variant in community wastewater—United States, November–December 2021. *Morbidity and Mortality Weekly Report* 71:103–105. https://doi.org/10.15585/mmwr.mm7103a5 (accessed May 10, 2024).

Klaassen, F., R. H. Holm, T. Smith, T. Cohen, A. Bhatnagar, and N. A. Menzies. 2024. Predictive power of wastewater for nowcasting infectious disease transmission: A retrospective case study of five sewershed areas in Louisville, Kentucky. *Environmental Research* 240(Pt 2):117395. https://doi.org/10.1016/j.envres.2023.117395 (accessed May 10, 2024).

Klevens, R. M., C. C. W. Young, S. W. Olesen, A. Osinski, D. Church, J. Muten, L. Chou, T. Segal, and K. Cranston. 2023. Evaluation of wastewater surveillance for SARS-CoV-2 in Massachusetts correctional facilities, 2020–2022. *Frontiers in Water* 5. https://doi.org/10.3389/frwa.2023.1083316 (accessed May 10, 2024).

Kmush, B. L., D. Monk, H. Green, D. A. Sachs, T. Zeng, and D. A. Larsen. 2022. Comparability of 24-hour composite and grab samples for detection of SARS-2-CoV RNA in wastewater. *FEMS Microbes* 3. https://doi.org/10.1093/femsmc/xtac017 (accessed May 10, 2024).

Kosulin, K., E. Geiger, A. Vecsei, W. D. Huber, M. Rauch, E. Brenner, F. Wrba, K. Hammer, A. Innerhofer, U. Potschger, A. Lawitschka, S. Matthes-Leodolter, G. Fritsch, and T. Lion. 2016. Persistence and reactivation of human adenoviruses in the gastrointestinal tract. *Clinical Microbiology and Infection* 22(4):381.e1–381.e8. https://doi.org/10.1016/j.cmi.2015.12.013 (accessed May 13, 2024).

Kralik, P., and M. Ricchi. 2017. A basic guide to real time PCR in microbial diagnostics: Definitions, parameters, and everything. *Frontiers in Microbiology* 8:108.

Kumblathan, T., Y. Liu, G. K. Uppal, S. E. Hrudey, and X.-F. Li. 2021. Wastewater-based epidemiology for community monitoring of SARS-CoV-2: Progress and challenges. *ACS Environmental Au* 1(1):18–31. https://doi.org/10.1021/acsenvironau.1c00015 (accessed May 13, 2024).

Lai, M., Y. Cao, S. S. Wulff, T. J. Robinson, A, McGuire, and B. Bisha. 2023. A time series based machine learning strategy for wastewater-based forecasting and nowcasting of COVID-19 dynamics. *Science of the Total Environment* 897:165105. https://doi.org/10.1016/j.scitotenv.2023.165105 (accessed May 13, 2024).

Langan, L. M., M. O'Brien, Z. C. Rundell, J. A. Black, B. J. Ryan, C. K. Chandliss, R. S. Norman, and B. W. Brooks. 2022. Comparative analysis of RNA-extraction approaches and associated influences on RT-qPCR of the SARS-CoV-2 RNA in a university residence hall and quarantine location. *ACS ES&T Water* 2(11):1929–1943. https://doi.org/10.1021/acsestwater.1c00476 (accessed May 13, 2024).

Langeveld, J., R. Schilperoot, L. Heijnen, G. Elsinga, C. E. M. Schapendonk, E. Fanoy, E. I. T. de Schepper, M. P. G. Koopmans, M. de Graaf, and G. Medema. 2023. Normalisation of SARS-CoV-2 concentrations in wastewater: The use of flow, electrical conductivity and crAssphage. *Science of the Total Environment* 865:161196. https://doi.org/10.1016/j.scitotenv.2022.161196 (accessed May 13, 2024).

Lanning, A., and E. W. Peterson. 2012. Evaluating subdivisions for identifying extraneous flow in separate sanitary sewer systems. *Journal of Water Resource and Protection* 4(6):334–341. https://doi.org/10.4236/jwarp.2012.46037 (accessed May 13, 2024).

Leisman, K. P., C. Owen, M. M. Warns, A. Tiwari, G. (Z). Bian, S. M. Owens, S. Catlett, A. Shrestha, R. Porestsky, A. I. Packman, and N. M. Mangan. 2024. A modeling pipeline to relate municipal wastewater surveillance and regional public health data. *Water Research* 252:121178. https://doi.org/10.1016/j.watres.2024.121178 (accessed May 13, 2024).

Lenaker, P., M. A. Pronschinske, S. R. Corsi, J. P. Stokdyk, H. T. Olds, D. K. Dila, and S. L. McLellan. 2024. A multi-marker assessment of sewage contamination in streams using human-associated indicator bacteria, human-specific viruses, and pharmaceuticals. *Science of the Total Environment* 930:172505. https://doi.org/10.1016/j.scitotenv.2024.172505 (accessed May 13, 2024).

Li, F., J. Deng, C. Xie, G. Wang, M. Xu, C. Wu, J. Li, and Y. Zhong. 2023. The differences in virus shedding time between the Delta variant and original SARS-CoV-2 infected patients. *Frontiers in Public Health* 11:1132643. https://doi.org/10.3389/fpubh.2023.1132643 (accessed May 13, 2024).

Li, J., W. Ahmed, S. Metcalfe, W. J. M. Smith, B. Tscharke, P. Lynch, S. Sherman, P. H. N. Vo, S. L. Kaserzan, S. L. Simpson, D. T. McCarthy, K. V. Thomas, J. F. Mueller, and P. Thai. 2022. Monitoring of SARS-CoV-2 in sewersheds with low COVID-19 cases using a passive sampling technique. *Water Research* 218:118481. https://doi.org/10.1016/j.watres.2022.118481 (accessed May 13, 2024).

Li, J., I. Hosegood, D. Powell, B. Tscharke, J. Lawler, K. V. Thomas, and J. F. Mueller. 2023. A global aircraft-based wastewater genomic surveillance network for early warning of future pandemics. *Lancet Global Health* 11(5):e791–e795. https://doi.org/10.1016/s2214-109x(23)00129-8 (accessed May 13, 2024).

Li, X., S. Zhang, S. Sherchan, G. Orive, U. Lertxundi, E. Haramoto, R. Honda, M. Kumar, S. Arora, M. Kitajima, and G. Jiang. 2023. Correlation between SARS-CoV-2 RNA concentration in wastewater and COVID-19 cases in community: A systematic review and meta-analysis. *Journal of Hazardous Materials* 441:129848. https://doi.org/10.1016/j.jhazmat.2022.129848 (accessed May 13, 2024).

Liu, P., M. Ibaraki, J. VanTassell, K. Geith, M. Cavallo, R. Kann, L. Guo, and C. L. Moe. 2022. A sensitive, simple, and low-cost method for COVID-19 wastewater surveillance at an institutional level. *Science of the Total Environment* 807:151047. https://doi.org/10.1016/j.scitotenv.2021.151047 (accessed May 13, 2024).

Liu, Y., W. Smith, M. Gebrewold, X. Wang, S. L. Simpson, A. Bivins, and W. Ahmed. 2023. Comparison of concentration and extraction workflows for qPCR quantification of intI1 and vanA in untreated wastewater. *Science of the Total Environment* 903:166442. https://doi.org/10.1016/j.scitotenv.2023.166442 (accessed May 13, 2024).

Maere, T., J. D. Therrien, and P. Vanrolleghem. 2022. *Normalization practices for SARS-CoV-2 data in wastewater-based epidemiology*. Quebec, Canada. Université Laval. https://nccid.ca/wp-content/uploads/sites/2/2023/02/Normalization-practices-Technical-Report-Final3.pdf (accessed May 13, 2024).

Markt, R., M. Mayr, E. Peer, A. O. Wagner, N. Lackner, and H. Insam. 2021. Detection and stability of SARS-CoV-2 fragments in wastewater: Impact of storage temperature. *Pathogens* 10(9):1215. https://doi.org/10.3390/pathogens10091215 (accessed May 13, 2024).

Martín-Pozo, L., M. del Carmen Gomez-Regalado, M. T. Garcia-Corcoles, and A. Zafra-Gomez. 2022. Chapter 16: Removal of quinolone antibiotics from wastewaters and sewage sludge. *Emerging contaminants in the environment* pp. 381–406. Amsterdam: Elsevier. https://doi.org/10.1016/B978-0-323-85160-2.00015-9 (accessed May 13, 2024).

McLellan, S. L., and A. Roguet. 2019. The unexpected habitat in sewer pipes for the propagation of microbial communities and their imprint on urban waters. *Current Opinion in Biotechnology* 57:34–41. https://doi.org/10.1016/j.copbio.2018.12.010 (accessed May 13, 2024).

Meadows, T., E. R. Coats, S. Narum, E. Top, B. J. Ridenhour, and T. Stalder. 2024. Epidemiological model can forecast COVID-19 outbreaks from wastewater-based surveillance in rural communities. *medRxiv.* https://doi.org/10.1101/2024.02.01.24302131 (accessed May 13, 2024).

Medema, G., L. Heijnen, G. Elsinga, R. Italiaander, and A. Brouwer. 2020. Presence of SARS-coronavirus-2 RNA in sewage and correlation with reported COVID-19 prevalence in the early stage of the epidemic in the Netherlands. *Environmental Science & Technology Letters* 7(7):511–516. https://doi.org/10.1021/acs.estlett.0c00357 (accessed May 13, 2024).

Mello, M. M., G. Triantis, R. Stanton, E. Blumenkranz, and D. M. Studdert. 2020. Waiting for data: Barriers to executing data use agreements. *Science* 367(6474):150–152. https://doi.org/10.1126/science.aaz7028 (accessed May 13, 2024).

Mello, M. M., J. S. Meschke, and G. H. Palmer. 2023. Mainstreaming wastewater surveillance for infectious disease. *The New England Journal of Medicine* 388(16):1441–1444.

Mercier, E., et al. 2022. Municipal and neighbourhood level wastewater surveillance and subtyping of an influenza virus outbreak. *Scientific Reports* 12(1):15777. https://doi.org/10.1038/s41598-022-20076-z (accessed May 13, 2024).

Metcalf & Eddy Inc., G. Tchobanoglous, F. L. Burton, R. Tsuchihashi, and H. D. Stensel. 2013. *Wastewater Engineering: Treatment and Resource Recovery*. McGraw-Hill.

Milne-Price, S., K. L. Miaszgowicz, and V. J. Munster. 2014. The emergence of the Middle East respiratory syndrome coronavirus. *Pathogens and Disease* 71(2):121–136. https://doi.org/10.1111/2049-632x.12166 (accessed May 13, 2024).

Monaghan, T. F., S. N. Rahman, C. W. Agudelo, A. J. Wein, J. M. Lazar, K. Everaert, and R. R. Dmochowski. 2021. Foundational statistical principles in medical research: Sensitivity, specificity, positive predictive value, and negative predictive value. *Medicina* 57(5):503. https://doi.org/10.3390/medicina57050503 (accessed May 13, 2024).

Mousa, A., et al. 2021. Social contact patterns and implications for infectious disease transmission—a systematic review and meta-analysis of contact surveys. *eLife* 10:e70294. https://doi.org/10.7554/eLife.70294 (accessed May 13, 2024).

Nadeau, S., et al. 2024. Influenza transmission dynamics quantified from RNA in wastewater in Switzerland. *Swiss Medical Weekly* 154(1):3503. https://doi.org/10.57187/s.3503 (accessed May 13, 2024).

NASEM (National Academies of Sciences, Engineering, and Medicine). 2023. *Wastewater-based disease surveillance for public health action.* Washington, DC: The National Academies Press. http://doi.org/10.17226/26767 (accessed June 17, 2024).

Nasir, J. A., et al. 2020. A comparison of whole genome sequencing of SARS-CoV-2 using amplicon-based sequencing, random hexamers, and bait capture. *Viruses* 12(8):895. https://doi.org/10.3390/v12080895 (accessed May 13, 2024).

Natarajan, A., et al. 2023. The tomato brown rugose fruit virus movement protein gene is a novel microbial source tracking marker. *Applied and Environmental Microbiology* 89(7). https://doi.org/10.1128/aem.00583-23 (accessed May 10, 2024).

Noble, R. T., S. M. Allen, A. D. Blackwood, W. Chu, S. C. Jiang, G. L. Lovelace, M. D. Sobsey, J. R. Stewart, and D. A. Wait. 2003. Use of viral pathogens and indicators to differentiate between human and non-human fecal contamination in a microbial source tracking comparison study. *Journal of Water and Health* 1(4):195–207. https://pubmed.ncbi.nlm.nih.gov/15382724/ (accessed April 1, 2024).

OMB (Office of Management and Budget). 2024. *Budget of the U.S. Government fiscal year 2025.* Washington, DC: Office of Management and Budget.

Otto, J. L., M. Holodniy, and R. F. DeFraites. 2014. Public health practice is not research. *American Journal of Public Health* 104(4):596–602. https://doi.org/10.2105/AJPH.2013.301663 (accessed May 13, 2024).

Parkins, M. D., B. E. Lee, N. Acosta, M. Bautista, C. R. J. Hubert, S. E. Hrudey, K. Frankowski, and X. Pang. 2023. Wastewater-based surveillance as a tool for public health action: SARS-CoV-2 and beyond. *Clinical Microbiology* 37(1):e00103-22. https://doi.org/10.1128/cmr.00103-22 (accessed June 4, 2024).

Parks, D. H., C. Rinke, M. Chuvochina, P.-A. Chaumeil, B. J. Woodcroft, P. N. Evans, P. Hugenholtz, and G. W. Tyson. 2017. Recovery of nearly 8,000 metagenome-assembled genomes substantially expands the tree of life. *Nature Microbiology* 2(11):1533–1542. https://doi.org/10.1038/s41564-017-0012-7 (accessed May 13, 2024).

Pecson, B. M., et al. 2021. Reproducibility and sensitivity of 36 methods to quantify the SARS-CoV-2 genetic signal in raw wastewater: Findings from an interlaboratory methods evaluation in the US. *Environmental Science: Water Research & Technology* 7(3):504–520. https://doi.org/10.1039/D0EW00946F (accessed May 13, 2024).

Pellegrinelli, L., C. Galli, A. Seiti, V. Primache, A. Hirvonen, S. Schiarea, G. Salmoiraghi, S. Castiglioni, E. Ammoni, D. Cereda, S. Binda, and E. Pariani. 2023. Wastewater-based epidemiology revealed in advance the increase of enterovirus circulation during the COVID-19 pandemic. *Science of the Total Environment* 902:166539. https://doi.org/10.1016/j.scitotenv.2023.166539 (accessed May 13, 2024).

Pérez-Cataluña, A., E. Cuevas-Ferrando, W. Randazzo, I. Falco, A. Allende, and G. Sanchez. 2021. Comparing analytical methods to detect SARS-CoV-2 in wastewater. *Science of the Total Environment* 758:143870. https://doi.org/10.1016/j.scitotenv.2020.143870 (accessed May 13, 2024).

Pérez-Zabaleta, M., C. Williams, and Z. Cetecioglu. 2022. New primer sets to detect recent human adenovirus F41 variants in wastewater: Is it linked to the new acute hepatitis? *medRxiv.* https://doi.org/10.1101/2022.09.16.22280038 (accessed May 13, 2024).

Phan, T., S. Brozak, B. Pell, A. Gitter, A. Xiao, K. D. Mena, Y. Kuang, and F. Wu. 2023. A simple SEIR-V model to estimate COVID-19 prevalence and predict SARS-CoV-2 transmission using wastewater-based surveillance data. *Science of the Total Environment* 857:159326. https://doi.org/10.1016/j.scitotenv.2022.159326 (accessed May 14, 2024).

Philo, S. E., E. K. Keim, R. Swanstrom, A. Q. W. Ong, E. A. Burnor, A. L. Kossik, J. C. Harrison, B. A. Demeke, N. A. Zhou, N. K. Beck, J. H. Shirai, and J. S. Meschke. 2021. A comparison of SARS-CoV-2 wastewater concentration methods for environmental surveillance. *Science of the Total Environment* 760:144215. https://doi.org/10.1016/j.scitotenv.2020.144215 (accessed July 24, 2024).

Piotrowska, M., D. Przygodzinska, K. Matyjewicz, and M. Popowska. 2017. Occurrence and variety of β-lactamase genes among *Aeromonas* spp. isolated from urban wastewater treatment plant. *Frontiers in Microbiology* 8:863. https://doi.org/10.3389/fmicb.2017.00863 (accessed May 13, 2024).

Polcz, P., K. Tornai, J. Juhász. G. Cserey, T. Pándics, E. Róka, M. Vargha, I. Z. Reguly, A. Csikász-Nagy, S. Pongor, and G. Szederkenyi. 2023. Wastewater-based modeling, reconstruction, and prediction for COVID-19 outbreaks in Hungary caused by highly immune evasive variants. *Water Research* 241:120098. https://doi.org/10.1016/j.watres.2023.120098 (accessed May 13, 2024).

Prasek, S. M., I. L. Pepper, G. K. Innes, S. Slinki, M. Ruedas, A. Sanchez, P. Bierly, W. Q. Betancourt, E. R. Stark, A. R. Foster, N. D. Betts-Childress, and B. W. Schmitz. 2022. Population level SARS-CoV-2 fecal shedding rates determined via wastewater-based epidemiology. *Science of the Total Environment* 838:156535. https://doi.org/10.1016/j.scitotenv.2022.156535 (accessed May 13, 2024).

Prasek, S. M., I. L. Pepper, G. K. Innes, S. Slinksi, W. Q. Betancourt, A. R. Foster, H. D. Yaglom, W. T. Porter, D. M. Engelthaler, and B. W. Schmitz. 2023. Variant-specific SARS-CoV-2 shedding rates in wastewater. *Science of the Total Environment* 857:159165. https://doi.org/10.1016/j.scitotenv.2022.159165 (accessed May 13, 2024).

Rainey, A. L., S. Liang, J. H. Bisesi, Jr., T. Sabo-Attwood, and A. T. Maurelli. 2023. A multistate assessment of population normalization factors for wastewater-based epidemiology of COVID-19. *PLoS One* 18(4):e0284370. https://doi.org/10.1371/journal.pone.0284370 (accessed May 13, 2024).

Ramuta, M. D., et al. 2022. SARS-CoV-2 and other respiratory pathogens are detected in continuous air samples from congregate settings. *Nature Communications* 13(1):4717. https://doi.org/10.1038/s41467-022-32406-w (accessed May 13, 2024).

Robinson, C. A., H. Y. Hsieh, S. Y. Hsu, Y. Wang, B. T. Salcedo, A. Blelenchia, J. Klutts, S. Zemmer, M. Reynolds, E. Semkiw, T. Foley, X. F. Wan, C. G. Wieberg, J. Wenzel, C. H. Lin, and M. C. Johnson. 2022. Defining biological and biophysical properties of SARS-CoV-2 genetic material in wastewater. *Science of The Total Environment* 807:150786.

Rodríguez, A., J. Cui, N. Ramakrishnan, B. Adhikari, and B. A. Prakash. 2023. EINNs: Epidemiologically-informed neural networks. *Proceedings of the AAAI Conference on Artificial Intelligence* 37(12):14453–14460. https://doi.org/10.1609/aaai.v37i12.26690 (accessed May 13, 2024).

Rodriguez-Mozaz, S., S. Chamorro, E. Marti, B. Huerta, M. Gros, A. Sanchez-Melsio, C. M. Borrego, D. Barceló, and J. L. Balcázar. 2015. Occurrence of antibiotics and antibiotic resistance genes in hospital and urban wastewaters and their impact on the receiving river. *Water Research* 69:234–242. https://doi.org/10.1016/j.watres.2014.11.021 (accessed May 13, 2024).

Ross, J. S., J. Waldstreicher, and H. M. Krumholz. 2023. Data sharing—a new era for research funded by the U.S. government. *New England Journal of Medicine* 389(26):2408–2410. https://www.nejm.org/doi/10.1056/NEJMp2308792 (accessed May 13, 2024).

Rossi, A., J. Chavez, T. Iverson, J. Hergert, K. Oakeson, N. LaCross, C. Njoku, A. Gorzalski, and D. Gerrity. 2023. *Candida auris* discovery through community wastewater surveillance during healthcare outbreak, Nevada, USA, 2022. *Emerging Infectious Diseases* 29(2). https://doi.org/10.3201/eid2902.221523 (accessed May 13, 2024).

Rusiñol, M., S. Martínez-Puchol, E. Forés, M. Itarte, R. Girones, and S. Bofill-Mas. 2020. Concentration methods for the quantification of coronavirus and other potentially pandemic enveloped virus from wastewater. *Current Opinion in Environmental Science & Health* 17:21-28. https://doi.org/10.1016/j.coesh.2020.08.002 (accessed July 24, 2024).

Salem, N., A. Mansour, M. Ciuffo, B. W, Falk, and M. Turina. 2015. A new tobamovirus infecting tomato crops in Jordan. *Archives of Virology* 161(2):503–506. https://doi.org/10.1007/s00705-015-2677-7 (accessed May 13, 2024).

Schang, C., et al. 2021. Passive sampling of SARS-CoV-2 for wastewater surveillance. *Environmental Science & Technology* 55(15):10432–10441. https://doi.org/10.1021/acs.est.1c01530 (accessed May 13, 2024).

Schneider, R., K. Weisbeck, K. Sheth, P. Sikes, L. Stadler, K. B. Ensor, R. Shaw, C. Berkobien, A. Wheeler, C. D. Johnson, C. Lengsfeld, and L. Hopkins. 2024. Assessment of public health agency and utility training needs for CDC National Wastewater Surveillance System jurisdictions in the United States. https://doi.org/10.1177/15248399241275617 (accessed November 20, 2024).

Schoen, M. E., M. K. Wolfe, L. Li, D. Duong, B. J. White, B. Hughes, and A. B. Boehm. 2022. SARS-CoV-2 RNA wastewater settled solids surveillance frequency and impact on predicted COVID-19 incidence using a distributed lag model. *ACS ES&T Water* 2(11):2167–2174. https://doi.org/10.1021/acsestwater.2c00074 (accessed May 13, 2024).

Schussman, M. K., and S. L. McLellan. 2022. Effect of time and temperature on SARS-CoV-2 in municipal wastewater conveyance systems. *Water* 14(9):1373. https://doi.org/10.3390/w14091373 (accessed May 13, 2024).

Schussman, M. K., A. Roguet, A. Schmoldt, B. Dinan, and S. L. McLellan. 2022. Wastewater surveillance using ddPCR accurately tracked Omicron emergence due to altered N1 probe binding efficiency. *Environmental Science: Water Research & Technology* 8(10):2190–2195. https://doi.org/10.1039/D2EW00194B (accessed May 13, 2024).

Servetas, S. L., K. H. Parratt, N. E. Brinkman, O. C. Shanks, T. Smith, P. J. Mattson, and N. J. Lin. 2022. Standards to support an enduring capability in wastewater surveillance for public health: Where are we? *Case Studies in Chemical and Environmental Engineering* 6:100247.

Sheth, K., L. Hopkins, K. Domakonda, L. Stadler, K. B. Ensor, C. D. Johnson, J. White, D. Persse, and E. Septimus. 2024a. Wastewater target pathogens of public health importance for expanded sampling, Houston, Texas, USA. *Emerging infectious diseases* 30(8):14–17. https://doi.org/10.3201/eid3008.231564 (accessed November 20, 2024).

Sheth, K., K. Domakonda, K. Short, L. Stadler, K. B. Ensor, C. D. Johnson, S. L. Williams, D. Pearse, and L. Hopkins. 2024b. A novel framework for internal responses to detection of pathogens in wastewater by public health agencies. *Public Health Reports*, p.00333549241253787.

Shum, E. Y., J. H. Lai, S. Li, H. G. Lee, J. Soliman, V. K. Raol, C. K. Lee, S. P. A. Fodor, and H. C. Fan. 2022. Next-generation digital polymerase chain reaction: High-dynamic-range single-molecule DNA counting via ultrapartitioning. *Analytical Chemistry* 94(51):17868–17876. https://doi.org/10.1021/acs.analchem.2c03649 (accessed May 13, 2024).

Sikorski, M. J., and M. M. Levine. 2020. Reviving the "Moore swab": A classic environmental surveillance tool involving filtration of flowing surface water and sewage water to recover typhoidal *Salmonella* bacteria. *Applied and Environmental Microbiology* 86(13). https://doi.org/10.1128/aem.00060-20 (accessed May 14, 2024).

Simpson, A., A. Topol, B. J. White, M. K. Wolfe, K. R. Wigginton, and A. B. Boehm. 2021. Effect of storage conditions on SARS-CoV-2 RNA quantification in wastewater solids. *PeerJ* 9:e11933. https://doi.org/10.7717/peerj.11933 (accessed May 14, 2024).

Sinton, L. W., R. K. Finlay, and D. J. Hannah. 1998. Distinguishing human from animal faecal contamination in water: A review. *New Zealand Journal of Marine and Freshwater Research* 32(2):323–348. https://doi.org/10.1080/00288330.1998.9516828 (accessed May 14, 2024).

Soloviev, K. 2016. *3 Steps to a Data-Driven Content Quality Approach.* Contentquo. https://www.contentquo.com/blog/3-steps-to-a-data-driven-content-quality-approach (accessed November 20, 2024).

Spaulding, A. C., L. B. Saber, S. Kennedy, Y. Yang, K. Moore, Y. Wang, S. P. Hilton, T. Chang, P. Liu, V. L. Phillips, M. J. Akiyama, and C. L. Moe. 2023. Wastewater surveillance for SARS-CoV-2 in an Atlanta, Georgia jail: A study of the feasibility of wastewater monitoring and correlation of building wastewater and individual testing results. *medRxiv.* https://doi.org/10.1101/2023.05.17.23290000 (accessed May 14, 2024).

Steele, J. A., A. G. Zimmer-Faust, J. F. Griffith, and S. B. Weisberg. 2021. Sources of variability in methods for processing, storing, and concentrating SARS-CoV-2 in influent from urban wastewater treatment plants. *medRxiv.* https://doi.org/10.1101/2021.06.16.21259063 (accessed May 14, 2024).

Stone, W., B.-L. Jones, J. Wilsenach, and A. Botha. 2012. External ecological niche for *Candida albicans* within reducing, oxygen-limited zones of wetlands. *Applied and Environmental Microbiology* 78(7).2443–2445. https://doi.org/10.1128/aem.06343-11 (accessed May 14, 2024).

Tanne, J. H. 2023. US expands testing of international air travellers to cover 30 respiratory viruses. *British Medical Journal* 383:2630. https://doi.org/10.1136/bmj.p2630 (accessed May 14, 2024).

Taylor, L. H., S. M. Latham, and M. E. J. Woolhouse. 2001. Risk factors for human disease emergence. *Philosophical Transactions of the Royal Society of London. Series B: Biological Sciences* 356(1411):983–989. https://doi.org/10.1098/rstb.2001.0888 (accessed May 14, 2024).

Tayoun, A., P. R. Burchard, A. M. Caliendo, A. Scherer, and G. J. Tsongalis. 2015. A multiplex PCR assay for the simultaneous detection of *Chlamydia trachomatis, Neisseria gonorrhoeae*, and *Trichomonas vaginalis. Experimental and Molecular Pathology* 98(2):214–218. https://doi.org/10.1016/j.yexmp.2015.01.011 (accessed May 14, 2024).

Tedcastle, A., T. Wilton, E. Pegg, D. Klapsa, E. Bujaki, R. Mate, M. Fritzsche, M. Majumdar, and J. Martin. 2022. Detection of enterovirus D68 in wastewater samples from the UK between July and November 2021. *Viruses* 14(1):143. https://doi.org/10.3390/v14010143 (accessed May 14, 2024).

Teunis, P., K. Takumi, and K. Shinagawa. 2004. Dose response for infection by *Escherichia coli* O157:H7 from outbreak data. *Risk Analysis* 24(2):401–407. https://doi.org/10.1111/j.0272-4332.2004.00441.x (accessed May 14, 2024).

Teunis, P. F. M., F. H. A. Shukhrie, H. Vennema, J. Bogerman, M. F. C. Beersma, and M. P. G. Koopmans. 2014. Shedding of norovirus in symptomatic and asymptomatic infections. *Epidemiology and Infection* 143(8):1710–1717. https://doi.org/10.1017/s095026881400274x (accessed May 14, 2024).

Tiwari, A., W. Ahmed, S. Oikarinen, S. P. Sherchan, A. Heikinheimo, G. Jiang, S. L. Simpson, J. Greaves, and A. Bivins. 2022. Application of digital PCR for public health-related water quality monitoring. *Science of the Total Environment* 837:155663.

Trujillo, M., K. Cheung, A. Gao, I. Hoxie, S. Kannoly, N. Kubota, K. M. San, D. S. Smyth, and J. J. Dennehy. 2021. Protocol for safe, affordable, and reproducible isolation and quantitation of SARS-CoV-2 RNA from wastewater. *PloS One* 16(9):e0257454. https://doi.org/10.1371/journal.pone.0257454 (accessed July 12, 2024).

Tyson, G. W., J. Chapman, P. Hugenholtz, E. E. Allen, R. J. Ram, P. M. Richardson, V. V. Solovyev, E. M. Rubin, D. S. Rokhsar, and J. F. Banfield. 2004. Community structure and metabolism through reconstruction of microbial genomes from the environment. *Nature* 428(6978):37–43. https://doi.org/10.1038/nature02340 (accessed May 14, 2024).

U.S. Census Bureau. 2022. *The 2021 American Housing Survey.* https://www.census.gov/programs-surveys/ahs/data/2021/ahs-2021-public-use-file--puf-/ahs-2021-national-publicuse-file--puf-.html (accessed May 14, 2024).

USDOT (U.S. Department of Transporation). 2024. *International Aviation Development Series: U.S. international air passenger and freight statistics.* Washington, DC: U.S. DOT.

Usmani, M., K. D. Brumfield, B. Magers, A. Zhou, C. Oh, Y. Mao, W. Brown, A. Schmidt, C.-Y. Wu, J. L. Shisler, T. H. Nguyen, A. Huq, R. Cowell, and A. Jutla. 2024. Building environmental and sociological predictive intelligence to understand the seasonal threat of SARS-CoV-2 in human populations. *American Journal of Tropical Medicine and Hygiene* 110(3):518–528. https://doi.org/10.4269/ajtmh.23-0077 (accessed May 14, 2024).

Uyeki, T. M., S. Milton, C. Abdul Hamid, C., Reinoso Webb, S. M. Presley, V. Shetty, S. N. Rollo, D. L. Martinez, S. Rai, E. R. Gonzales, K. L. Kniss, Y. Jang, J. C. Frederick, J. A. De La Cruz, J. Liddell, H. Di, M. K. Kirby, J. R. Barnes, and C. T. Davis. 2024. Highly pathogenic avian influenza A(H5N1) virus infection in a dairy farm worker. *New England Journal of Medicine* 390(21):2028–2029. https://doi.org/10.1056/NEJMc2405371 (accessed May 14, 2024).

Vaughan, L., M. Zhang, H. Gu, J. B. Rose, C. C. Naughton, G. Medema, V. Allan, A. Roiko, L. Blackhall, and A. Zanyadi. 2023. An exploration of challenges associated with machine learning for time series forecasting of COVID-19 community spread using wastewater-based epidemiological data. *Science of the Total Environment* 858(Pt 1):159748. https://doi.org/10.1016/j.scitotenv.2022.159748 (accessed May 14, 2024).

Velappan, N., K. Davis-Anderson, and A. Deshpande. 2022. Warning signs of potential black swan outbreaks in infectious disease. *Frontiers in Microbiology* 13. https://doi.org/10.3389/fmicb.2022.845572 (accessed May 14, 2024).

Wade, M. J., A. L. Jacomo, E. Armenise, M. R. Brown, J. T. Bunce, G. J. Cameron, Z. Fang, D. F. Gilpin, D. W. Graham, J. M. Grimsley, and A. Hart. 2022. Understanding and managing uncertainty and variability for wastewater monitoring beyond the pandemic: Lessons learned from the United Kingdom national COVID-19 surveillance programmes. *Journal of Hazardous Materials* 424:127456.

WEF (Water Environment Federation). 2021. *Safety, health, and security standards for water resource recovery, Manual of practice No. 1,* 7th Edition. WEF Press. Alexandria, Virginia. 416 p.

Wegrzyn, R. D., G. D. Appiah, R. Morfino, S. R. Milford, A. T. Walker, E. T. Ernst, W. W. Darrow, S. L. Li, K. Robinson, D. MacCannell, D. Dai, B. P. Girinthian, A. L. Hicks, B. Cosca, G. Woronoff, A. M. Plocik, B. P. Girinathan, L. Moriarty, S. A. J. Guagliardo, M. S. Cetron, and C. R. Friedman. 2023. Early detection of severe acute respiratory syndrome coronavirus 2 variants using traveler-based genomic surveillance at 4 US airports, September 2021–January 2022. *Clinical Infectious Diseases* 76(3):e540–e543. https://doi.org/10.1093/cid/ciac461 (accessed May 14, 2024).

Weil, M., M. Mandelboim, E. Mendelson, Y. Manor, L. Shulman, D. Ram, G. Barkai, Y. Shemer, D. Wolf, Z. Kra-oz, L. Weiss, R. Pando, M. Hindiyeh, and D. Sofer. 2017. Human enterovirus D68 in clinical and sewage samples in Israel. *Journal of Clinical Virology* 86:52–55. https://doi.org/10.1016/j.jcv.2016.11.013 (accessed May 14, 2024).

Whitney, O. N., L. C. Kennedy, V. B. Fan, A. Hinkle, R. Kantor, H. Greenwald, A. Crits-Christoph, B. Al-Sayeb, M. Chaplin, A. C. Maurer, R. Tijan, and K. L. Nelson. 2021. Sewage, salt, silica, and SARS-CoV-2 (4S): An economical kit-free method for direct capture of SARS-CoV-2 RNA from wastewater. *Environmental Science & Technology* 55(8):4880–4888. https://doi.org/10.1021/acs.est.0c08129 (accessed May 14, 2024).

Wilde, H., W. B. Perry, O. Jones, P. Kille, A. Weightman, D. L. Jones, G. Cross, and I. Durance. 2022. Accounting for dilution of SARS-CoV-2 in wastewater samples using physicochemical markers. *Water* 14(18):2885.

WHO (World Health Organization). 2024. *Laboratory biosafety guidance related to SARS-CoV-2 (COVID-19).* https://iris.who.int/bitstream/handle/10665/376231/WHO-WHE-EPP-2024.3-eng.pdf?sequence=1 (accessed May 14, 2024).

Woerther, P.-L., C. Burdet, E. Chachaty, and A. Andremont. 2013. Trends in human fecal carriage of extended-spectrum β-lactamases in the community: Toward the globalization of CTX-M. *Clinical Microbiology Reviews* 26(4):744–758. https://doi.org/10.1128/CMR.00023-13 (accessed May 14, 2024).

Wolfe, M. K., A. Topol, A. Knudson, A. Simpson, B. White, D. J. Vugia, A. T. Yu, L. Li, M. Balliet, P. Stoddard, G. S. Han, K. R. Wigginton, and A. B. Boehm. 2021. High-frequency, high-throughput quantification of SARS-CoV-2 RNA in wastewater settled solids at eight publicly owned treatment works in Northern California shows strong association with COVID-19 incidence. *mSystems* 6(5). https://doi.org/10.1128/msystems.00829-21 (accessed June 28, 2024).

Wolfe, M. K., D. Duong, K. M. Bakker, M. Ammerman, L. Mortenson, B. Hughes, P. Arts, A. S. Laurig, W. J. Fitzsimmons, E. Bendall, C. E. Hwang, E. T. Martin, B. J. White, A. B. Boehm, and K. R. Wigginton. 2022. Wastewater-based detection of two influenza outbreaks. *Environmental Science & Technology Letters* 9(8):687–692. https://doi.org/10.1021/acs.estlett.2c00350 (accessed May 14, 2024).

Wolfe, M. K., A. T. Yu, D. Duong, M. S. Rane, B. Hughes, V. Chan-Herur, M. Donnelly, S. Chai, B. J. White, D. J. Vugia, and A. B. Boehm. 2023. Use of wastewater for mpox outbreak surveillance in California. *The New England Journal of Medicine* 388(6):570–572. https://doi.org/10.1056/nejmc2213882 (accessed May 14, 2024).

Wolfe, M. K., A. H. Paulos, A. Zulli, D. Duong, B. Sheldon, B. J. White, and A. B. Boehm. 2024. Wastewater detection of emerging Arbovirus infections: Case study of dengue in the United States. *Environmental Science and Technology Letters* 11(1):9–15. https://doi.org/10.1021/acs.estlett.3c00769 (accessed May 14, 2024).

Wolfe, M. K., D. Duoung, B. Shelden, E. M. G. Chan, V. Chan-herur, S. Hilton, A. H. Paulos, X. R. S. Xu, A. Zulli, B. J. White, and A. B. Boehm. 2024b. Detection of hemagglutinin H5 influenza A virus sequence in municipal wastewater solids at wastewater treatment plants with increases in influenza A in spring, 2024. *Environmental Science & Technology Letters* 11(6):526-532.

Wolken, M., T. Sun, C. McCall, R. Schneider, K. Caton, C. Hundley, L. Hopkins, K. Endsor, K. Domakonda, P. Kalvapalle, D. Persse, S. Williams, and L. B. Stadler. 2023.Wastewater surveillance of SARS-CoV-2 and influenza in preK-12 schools shows school, community, and citywide infections. *Water Research.* https://doi.org/10.1016/j.watres.2023.119648 (accessed May 14, 2024).

Wollants, E., E. Keyaerts, L. Cuypers, M. Bloemen, M. Thijssen, S. Ombelet, J. Raymenants, K. Beuselinck, L. Laenen, L. Budts, B. Pussig, K. Lagrou, M. V. Ranst, and E. Andre. 2022. Environmental circulation of adenovirus 40/41 and SARS-CoV-2 in the context of the emergence of acute hepatitis of unknown origin. *medRxiv.* https://doi.org/10.1101/2022.06.08.22276091 (accessed May 14, 2024).

The Water Research Foundation. 2020. *Wastewater surveillance of the COVID-19 genetic signal in sewersheds recommendations from global experts.* Alexandria, VA: The Water Research Foundation. https://www.waterrf.org/sites/default/files/file/2020-06/COVID-19_SummitHandout-v3b.pdf (accessed April 16, 2024).

Yan, T., P. O'Brien, J. M. Shelton, A. C. Whelen, and E. Pagaling. 2018. Municipal wastewater as a microbial surveillance platform for enteric diseases: A case study for *Salmonella* and salmonellosis. *Environmental Science & Technology* 52(8):4869–4877. https://doi.org/10.1021/acs.est.8b00163 (accessed May 14, 2024).

Ye, Y., R. M. Ellenberg, K. E. Graham, and K. R. Wigginton. 2016. Survivability, partitioning, and recovery of enveloped viruses in untreated municipal wastewater. *Environmental Science & Technology* 50(10):5077–5085. https://doi.org/10.1021/acs.est.6b00876 (accessed May 14, 2024).

Yu, Q., S. W. Olesen, C. Duvallet, and Y. H. Grad. 2024. Assessment of sewer connectivity in the United States and its implications for equity in wastewater-based epidemiology. *medRxiv.* https://doi.org/10.1101/2023.05.24.23290486 (accessed May 14, 2024).

Zahedi, A., P. Monis, D. Deere, and U. Ryan. 2021. Wastewater-based epidemiology—surveillance and early detection of waterborne pathogens with a focus on SARS-CoV-2, Cryptosporidium and Giardia. *Parasitology Research* 120(12):4167-4188. https://doi.org/10.1007/s00436-020-07023-5 (accessed July 24, 2024).

Zambrana, W., C. Huang, D. Solis, M. K. Sahoo, B. A. Pinsky, and A. B. Boehm. 2024. Spatial and temporal variation in respiratory syncytial virus (RSV) subtype RNA in wastewater and relation to clinical specimens. *mSphere* 0:e00224-24.

Zhang, L., F. Chen, Z. Zeng, M. Xu, F. Sun, L. Yang, X. Bi, Y. Lin, Y. Gao, H. Hao, W. Yi, M. Li, and X. Xie. 2021. Advances in metagenomics and its application in environmental microorganisms. *Frontiers in Microbiology* 12. https://doi.org/10.3389/fmicb.2021.766364 (accessed May 14, 2024).

Zhang, S., J. Shi, X. Li, L. Coin, J. W. O'Brien, M. Sivakumar, F. Hai, and G. Jiang. 2023a. Triplex qPCR assay for *Campylobacter jejuni* and *Campylobacter coli* monitoring in wastewater. *Science of the Total Environment* 892:164574. https://doi.org/10.1016/j.scitotenv.2023.164574 (accessed May 14, 2024).

Zhang, S., J. Shi, E. Sharma, X. Li, S. Gao, X. Zhou, J. O'Brien, L. Coin, Y. Liu, M. Sivakumar, F. Hai, and G. Jiang. 2023b. In-sewer decay and partitioning of *Campylobacter jejuni* and *Campylobacter coli* and implications for their wastewater surveillance. *Water Research* 233:119737. https://doi.org/10.1016/j.watres.2023.119737 (accessed May 14, 2024).

Zhao, C., B. Dimitrov, M. Goldman, S. Nayfach, and K. S. Pollard. 2022. MIDAS2: Metagenomic Intra-species Diversity Analysis System. *Bioinformatics* 39(1). https://doi.org/10.1093/bioinformatics/btac713 (accessed May 14, 2024).

Zheng, S., et al. 2020. Viral load dynamics and disease severity in patients infected with SARS-CoV-2 in Zhejiang province, China, January-March 2020: Retrospective cohort study. *British Medical Journal* 369:m1443. https://doi.org/doi:10.1136/bmj.m1443 (accessed May 14, 2024).

Zheng, X., K. Zhao, X. Xu, Y. Deng, L. Leung, J. T. Wu, G. M. Leung, M. Peiris, L. L. M. Poon, and T. Zhang. 2023. Development and application of influenza virus wastewater surveillance in Hong Kong. *Water Research* 245:120594. https://doi.org/10.1016/j.watres.2023.120594 (accessed November 20, 2024).

Zulli, A., M. R. Varkila, J. Parsonnet, M. K. Wolfe, and A. B. Boehm. 2024. Observations of Respiratory Syncytial Virus (RSV) nucleic acids in wastewater solids across the United States in the 2022–2023 season: Relationships with RSV infection positivity and hospitalization rates. *ACS ES&T Water* 4(4):1657-1667. https://doi.org/10.1021/acsestwater.3c00725 (accessed July 12, 2024).

Appendix

Committee Members and Staff Biographical Sketches

COMMITTEE MEMBERS

Guy H. Palmer (NAM), *Chair,* holds the Jan and Jack Creighton Endowed Chair at Washington State University (WSU) where he is Regents Professor of Pathology & Infectious Diseases. The founding director of WSU's Paul G. Allen School for Global Health, he leads interdisciplinary health research as the senior director of global health. Dr. Palmer also holds adjunct appointments with the University of Nairobi, Kansas State University, and the Universidad del Valle de Guatemala. Dr. Palmer is a member of the National Academy of Medicine, a Medical Sciences Fellow of the American Association for the Advancement of Science, a Fellow of the American Academy of Microbiology, and a founding member of the Washington State Academy of Sciences, and currently serves on the Council for the National Institute of Allergy and Infectious Disease at the National Institutes of Health. He previously served as chair of the National Academies of Sciences, Engineering, and Medicine's Committee on Examining the Long-Term Health and Economic Effects of Antimicrobial Resistance in the United States. Dr. Palmer earned his Ph.D. in infectious diseases from WSU, and his B.S. in biology and a D.V.M. from Kansas State University. He holds honorary doctorates from the University of Bern (Dr. Med. Vet., 2011) and Kansas State University (Ph.D., 2016).

Ami S. Bhatt is an associate professor at Stanford University in the Departments of Medicine (Hematology; Blood & Marrow Transplantation) and Genetics. She is a physician scientist with a strong interest in microbial genomics and metagenomics. Her team's research program seeks to illuminate the interplay between the microbial environment and host/clinical factors in human diseases by developing and applying novel molecular and computational tools to study strain-level dynamics of the microbiome, to understand how microbial genomes change over time, and to predict the functional output of microbiomes. She is applying these tools to support wastewater-based disease surveillance in the San Francisco Bay area, both for COVID-19 as well as emerging disease. Dr. Bhatt has received multiple awards, including the Chen Award of Excellence from the Human Genome Organisation and the Sloan Foundation Fellowship; she is also an elected member of the American Society of Clinical Investigation. Dr. Bhatt co-founded the nonprofit Global Oncology and serves as the director for global oncology for Stanford's Center for Innovation in Global Health. She received her M.D. and Ph.D. from the University of California, San Francisco, followed by residency, fellowship, chief residency, and a postdoctoral fellowship at Harvard Medical School.

Marisa C. Eisenberg is a professor of epidemiology, complex systems, and mathematics at the University of Michigan, and the current director of the Center for the Study of Complex Systems. Her research is in mathematical epidemiology and infectious disease modeling, and blends mathematics, statistics, and epidemiology to understand transmission dynamics, inform intervention strategies, and improve forecasting. Her research includes a range of modeling and analysis of wastewater surveillance for infectious diseases, including polio, SARS-CoV-2, and other pathogens. During the pandemic, Dr. Eisenberg was closely involved in COVID-19 response efforts at both the state and university levels, developing modeling, analysis, and tools to understand COVID-19 in Michigan, for which she was recently awarded the University of Michigan's President's Award for National and State Leadership. Dr. Eisenberg received her M.S. and Ph.D. in biomedical engineering from the University of California, Los Angeles, and was a postdoctoral fellow at the Mathematical Biosciences Institute at Ohio State University.

Dr. Eisenberg receives U.S. Centers for Disease Control and Prevention Epidemiology and Laboratory Capacity for Prevention and Control of Emerging Infectious Disease funding via the Michigan Department of Health and Human Services to support the state's COVID-19 wastewater surveillance program. Dr. Eisenberg has made public statements regarding the use of wastewater surveillance as a key tool to assess disease beyond COVID-19, including polio.

Raul A. Gonzalez is the co-founder and principal scientist at H2O Molecular, bringing over fifteen years of experience in applying advanced molecular methods to water systems and related infrastructure. Prior to founding H2O Molecular, Dr. Gonzalez served as an environmental scientist at Hampton Roads Sanitation District (HRSD), where he led the molecular pathogen program for a decade. His work encompassed both molecular laboratory operations and field research, focusing on pathogen detection and surveillance. During the COVID-19 pandemic, Dr. Gonzalez played a pivotal role in expanding HRSD's research and laboratory capabilities, pioneering new methodologies for wastewater-based disease surveillance. His work also included use of nucleic acid–based markers for diverse applications, such as identifying compromised sewer infrastructure and assessing pathogen removal across various treatment processes. Dr. Gonzalez earned his B.S. in biology from the University of California, Los Angeles, and his Ph.D. in environmental science and engineering from the University of North Carolina at Chapel Hill.

Charles N. Haas (NAE) is the L.D. Betz Professor of Environmental Engineering at Drexel University, where he has been since 1991. From 2005 to 2020, he was also head of the Department of Civil, Architectural & Environmental Engineering. For more than 35 years, Professor Haas has specialized in the assessment of risk from and control of human exposure to pathogenic microorganisms and, in particular, the treatment of water and wastewater to minimize microbial risk to human health. He co-directed the U.S. Environmental Protection Agency/U.S. Department of Homeland Security University Cooperative Center of Excellence–Center for Advancing Microbial Risk Assessment. He is a member of the National Academy of Engineering, a Board Certified Environmental Engineering Member by eminence of the American Academy of Environmental Engineers, and a fellow of the American Academy for the Advancement of Science and the American Academy of Microbiology. He has previously served on numerous National Academies of Sciences, Engineering, and Medicine committees, including the Committee on Strategies for Identifying and Addressing Vulnerabilities Posed by Synthetic Biology and planning committees for two symposia on gain of function research with H5N1/H7N9 avian influenza. He received his B.S. in biology and his M.S. in environmental engineering from the Illinois Institute of Technology, and his Ph.D. in environmental engineering from the University of Illinois at Urbana-Champaign.

Loren P. Hopkins is the chief environmental science officer at the City of Houston, chief of the Bureau of Community and Children's Environmental Health at the Houston Health Department, and a professor of practice in the Department of Statistics at Rice University. In this capacity, she conducts applied environmental health research and uses the results to inform policies at the City of Houston to improve the health of the community. In May 2020, Dr. Hopkins established a critical wastewater surveillance program at the Houston Health Department that continues to serve as a barometer on the spatiotemporal prevalence of the SARS-CoV-2 virus in the City of Houston. The SARS-CoV-2 wastewater surveillance sampling results have informed public health intervention decisions and aided in improving the response to the COVID-19 pandemic in Houston. She received the 2016 Teaching and Mentoring Award from the Graduate Student Association at Rice University. She holds a B.S. in geological sciences with emphasis in geophysics from the University of Texas at Austin and an M.S. and Ph.D. in environmental science and engineering from Rice University.

Dr. Hopkins is also serving as a paid consultant via StatAnalytics IDD LLC through June 2022 to support work on a U.S. Centers for Disease Control and Prevention Foundation–funded project on best practices in wastewater surveillance. In her capacity as the chief environmental science officer for the City of Houston, Dr. Hopkins has made public statements explaining how the city uses wastewater-based disease surveillance to inform its health initiatives.

Na'Taki Osborne Jelks is assistant professor of Environmental and Health Sciences and Director of the Sustainable Black Futures Lab at Spelman College in Atlanta, Georgia, and co-founder of the West Atlanta Watershed Alliance, a community-based environmental justice organization. In her research, Jelks champions community science and other participatory research approaches; she trains community residents to be watershed researchers who monitor water quality and investigate local environmental conditions, giving them actionable data to press for solutions to urban watershed and community health challenges. In 2021, Dr. Jelks was named an Ecological Society of America Excellence in Ecology Scholar. Since 2018, Jelks has served on the National Environmental Justice Advisory Council, a federal advisory committee that works to integrate environmental justice into the U.S. Environmental Protection Agency's programs, policies, and activities as well as to improve the environment or public health in communities disproportionately burdened by environmental harms and risks. Dr. Jelks holds a B.S. in chemistry and civil engineering from Spelman College and the Georgia Institute of Technology, an M.P.H. in environmental and occupational health from Emory University, and a Ph.D. in public health from Georgia State University.

Christine K. Johnson (NAM) is professor of epidemiology and ecosystem health and director of the EpiCenter for Disease Dynamics at the One Health Institute, University of California, Davis. Her work is committed to transdisciplinary research to characterize impacts of environmental change on animal and human health, inform preparedness for emerging threats, and guide public policy at the intersection of emerging disease and environmental health. Professor Johnson's research pioneers new approaches to characterization of emerging threats and disease dynamics at the animal-human interface in rapidly changing landscapes that constitute "fault lines" for disease emergence, disease spillover, and subsequent spread. She leads the EpiCenter for Emerging Infectious Disease Intelligence, one of the National Institute of Allergy and Infectious Diseases' Centers for Emerging Infectious Disease, to investigate the environment and climate-related drivers for spillover and spread of emerging ebolaviruses, coronaviruses, and arboviruses. She is a member of the National Academy of Medicine and was awarded the Distinguished Scholarly Public Service Award. She earned a B.S. in zoology and political science from Duke University; a Ph.D. in epidemiology from the University of California, Davis; and a V.M.D. degree in veterinary medicine from the University of Pennsylvania.

Rob Knight is the founding director of the Center for Microbiome Innovation and professor of pediatrics, bioengineering, and computer science and engineering at the University of California, San Diego. His research has linked microbes to a range of health conditions, enhanced our understanding of microbes in many environments, and made high-throughput sequencing accessible to thousands of researchers around the world. His laboratory has produced many of the software tools and laboratory techniques that enabled high throughput microbiome science, including QIIME and Uni-Frac. He is co-founder of the Earth Microbiome Project; the American Gut Project; and the company Biota, Inc., which uses deoxyribonucleic acid from microbes in the subsurface to guide oilfield decisions. He set up and runs the wastewater COVID-19 detection program and co-founded the COVID-19 testing laboratory at the University of California, San Diego, which performs thousands of clinical tests per day and also sequences viral genomes out of wastewater and clinical samples. He is a fellow of the American Association for the Advancement of Science and the American Academy of Microbiology and received the 2019 National Institutes of Health Director's Pioneer Award and 2017 Massry Prize. Dr. Knight earned his B.S. in biochemistry from the University of Otago and his Ph.D. in evolutionary biology from Princeton University.

Sandra L. McLellan is professor in the School of Freshwater Sciences at the University of Wisconsin-Milwaukee. Dr. McLellan's research program studies the human health relevance of microorganisms that flux between the primary habitat of human hosts and environmental reservoirs. Her research has identified new indicators of waterborne disease by characterizing the microbial population structure of sewage and also uses genomics and metagenomics to explore the unique microbiome of urban water infra-structure to understand the complex interactions within the community. Dr. McLellan currently works with the Wisconsin State Laboratory of Hygiene to conduct a statewide SARS-CoV-2 wastewater monitoring program. Dr. McLellan is a fellow in the American Academy of Microbiology and is a member of the International Water Association and the International Society for Microbiology. She received her B.S. in health sciences from the University of Wisconsin-Milwaukee and Ph.D. from the University of Cin-cinnati College of Medicine in environmental health.

Dr. McLellan receives U.S. Centers for Disease Control and Preven-tion Epidemiology and Laboratory Capacity for Prevention and Control of Emerging Infectious Disease funding via the Wisconsin Department of Health Services to support the state's COVID-19 wastewater surveillance program.

Michelle M. Mello (NAM) is professor of law at Stanford Law School and professor of health policy at Stanford University School of Medicine. She conducts empirical research into issues at the intersection of law, ethics, and health policy, with a focus on understanding the effects of law and regula-tion on healthcare delivery and population health outcomes. Her research interests include medical liability, public health law, pharmaceuticals and vaccines, biomedical research ethics and governance, and health informa-tion privacy. Dr. Mello received the Alice S. Hersh New Investigator Award from AcademyHealth, a Greenwall Faculty Scholars Award in Bioethics, and a Robert Wood Johnson Foundation Investigator Award in Health Policy Research and is a member of the National Academy of Medicine. She holds B.A.s in political science and applied ethics from Stanford University; an M.Phil. in comparative social research from Oxford University, where she was a Marshall Scholar; a J.D. from the Yale Law School; and a Ph.D. in health policy and administration from the University of North Carolina at Chapel Hill.

John Scott Meschke is professor and associate chair in the Department of Environmental and Occupational Health Sciences in the School of Public Health at the University of Washington. He is also an adjunct professor in civil and environmental engineering at the University of Washington. Dr. Meschke is an environmental and occupational health microbiologist and virologist specializing in the fate, transport, detection, and control of pathogens in environmental media. Over the past 10 years, his research has focused on development, validation, and implementation of wastewater sur-veillance methods for poliovirus, *Salmonella* Typhi, SARS-CoV-2, and other pathogens. Dr. Meschke recently served as a paid consultant to PATH (an international nongovernmental organization) on wastewater surveillance in developing countries and in an unpaid advisory role to the Washington State Department of Health to advise on wastewater surveillance methods in state correctional facilities. Dr. Meschke completed his B.S. in biology and J.D. at the University of Kansas, his M.S. in environmental science at Indiana University, and his Ph.D. in environmental sciences and engineering at the University of North Carolina at Chapel Hill.

During the timeframe of this study, Dr. Meschke received U.S. Centers for Disease Control and Prevention Epidemiology and Laboratory Capacity for Prevention and Control of Emerging Infectious Disease funding, as a subject matter expert, via the Washington State Department of Health to support the state's COVID-19 wastewater surveillance program. Dr. Meschke received donated supplies from Qiagen, Ceres Nano, and Macherey Nagel to evaluate wastewater surveillance products for SARS-CoV-2 without restrictions on the conduct of the research or the publication of the results.

Rekha Singh is a Biodefense Fellow at the Department of Defense working in support of the National Biodefense Strategy. Previously, she served as the wastewater surveillance program manager for the Virginia Department of Health, where she partnered with wastewater treatment plants, laboratories, and local health departments to design and implement the wastewater surveillance program for Virginia. Prior to this, she co-led the State Testing Task Force for pandemic response and led the establishment of the OneLab program to enhance testing in the Commonwealth of Virginia. She has a background in epidemiology, environmental health, contaminants remediation, disease surveillance, water and wastewater, community engagement, the development of novel point-of-use drinking water treatment technologies, and the deployment of these technologies in the real world. Dr. Singh earned a Ph.D. in environmental science and engineering with a focus on environmental health and an M.P.H. in health policy law and ethics from the University of Virginia.

Krista Wigginton is professor of environmental engineering and an associate department chair in the Department of Civil and Environmental Engineering at the University of Michigan. Her research team focuses on viruses in the environment, including their mechanistic fate, the role they play in urban water microbial ecology, and the development of novel detection methods. Prior to COVID-19, her team published studies on how coronaviruses behave in municipal wastewater and through water treatment processes and developed methods for recovering them from water samples. During the COVID-19 pandemic, she collaborated on a number of projects focused on implementing wastewater-based epidemiology programs. She is the recipient of a National Science Foundation CAREER Award and the Water Research Foundation Paul L. Busch Award. Dr. Wigginton received her B.S. in chemistry from the University of Idaho, and M.S. and Ph.D. in environmental engineering from Virginia Tech.

During the timeframe of this study, Dr. Wigginton worked on a U.S. Centers for Disease Control and Prevention (CDC) Foundation–funded project with Verily Life Sciences to demonstrate how to conduct and report wastewater-based disease surveillance. Dr. Wigginton receives CDC Epidemiology and Laboratory Capacity for Prevention and Control of Emerging Infectious Disease funding via the Michigan Department of Health and Human Services to support the state's COVID-19 wastewater surveillance program.

STUDY STAFF

Stephanie E. Johnson, *Study Director*, is a senior program officer with the Water Science and Technology Board. Since joining the National Research Council in 2002, she has worked on a wide range of water-related studies, on topics such as desalination, wastewater reuse, contaminant source remediation, coal and metal mining, coastal risk reduction, and ecosystem restoration. Dr. Johnson received her B.A. from Vanderbilt University in chemistry and geology and her M.S. and Ph.D. in environmental sciences from the University of Virginia.

Samuel Kraft is a senior program assistant with the Water Science and Technology Board and Board on Earth Sciences and Resources. Prior to joining the National Academies in April 2024, Sam worked as a ground penetrating radar analyst for a company that specializes in concrete services. Sam received his B.A. in geology from Millersville University of Pennsylvania.

Miles Lansing is a senior program assistant supporting the Water Science and Technology Board and Board on Earth Sciences and Resources in the Division on Earth and Life Studies. He received his B.A. from the University of Pittsburgh in political science in 2021, and has been with the National Academies of Sciences, Engineering, and Medicine for more than two years.